Aids to
Clinical Haematology

J. A. Child
MD FRCP
Consultant Clinical Haematologist and Physician
The General Infirmary at Leeds, Leeds, UK

A. C. Cuthbert
MRCP MRCPath
Consultant Haematologist
Airedale General Hospital, Keighley, UK

Second Edition

CHURCHILL LIVINGSTONE
EDINBURGH LONDON MADRID MELBOURNE NEW YORK AND TOKYO 1992

CHURCHILL LIVINGSTONE
Medical Division of Longman Group UK Limited

Distributed in the United States of America by
Churchill Livingstone Inc., 650 Avenue of the
Americas, New York, N.Y. 10011, and by associated
companies, branches and representatives
throughout the world.

First edition 1982
Second edition 1992

ISBN 0-443-04192 X

**British Library of Cataloguing in Publication
Data**
A catalogue record for this book is available from
the British Library.

**Library of Congress Cataloging in
Publication Data**
A catalog record for this book is available from the
Library of Congress.

The
publisher's
policy is to use
**paper manufactured
from sustainable forests**

Produced by Longman Singapore Publishers (Pte) Ltd
Printed in Singapore

Preface

The importance of haematology as a major subspecialty within clinical medicine is reflected in examinations at undergraduate and postgraduate levels. Knowledge of the subject is of value to a wide range of doctors and scientists, and developments in haematology, especially in relation to the haematological malignancies, continue to be at the leading edge of advances in medicine.

The format of this book, in the well-established 'Aids' series, is intended to provide a synoptic and yet reasonably comprehensive presentation of the subject. In a clinically orientated presentation it is often necessary to qualify information in order to convey its relative importance in practice. Equally, rare disorders have to be described in order to give the overall picture of the spectrum and interrelationships of disease states. The results of recent scientific advances should also be incorporated, particularly where this makes for easier understanding. Following these tenets, we have given the undergraduate more than the bare facts required for examinations. For the qualified doctor this book should serve as an easily accessible guide to use in practice and for the MRCP or MRCPath candidate an up-to-date distillation of the subject to use as a revision aid. It is hoped that non-medical scientists and health care workers, particularly specialist nurses, may also find the book useful for reference.

This second edition of *Aids to Clinical Haematology* takes account of recent advances and reflects newer perspectives, as for example in the lymphoproliferative diseases. There has been revision of many of the sections with the addition of new material including illustrations and tables. There are new sections on bone marrow transplantation, thrombosis and anticoagulation. As before, each disease or disorder is dealt with systematically—basic aetiological and pathological aspects preceding laboratory findings, which are in turn followed by clinical features, treatment and where relevant, course and prognosis. Chapters 19–24 provide background information and some of the basic 'shorthand' of haematology—morphological terminology and indices.

An index is provided. Suggestions for further, advanced reading are given (of more relevance to the MRCP or MRCPath candidate), with a list of standard textbooks in addition to recommended specialist journals and reviews.

Leeds 1992   J. A. Child

Contents

1. Iron deficiency anaemia

Basic nutritional features and metabolism of iron

1. Dietary iron
(i) Most important sources are red meats and liver. Some vegetables, e.g. pulses, are rich in iron
(ii) Mainly in ferric form and usually complexed
(iii) Daily iron requirements vary greatly according to age and sex—12 mg/day *minimum* recommended in adults (may be inadequate in females of reproductive age)

2. Absorption
(i) Preliminary release of ferric compounds from complexes and reduction to ferrous forms in the stomach
(ii) Mainly absorbed in the duodenum and first part of the jejunum
(iii) Generally an inverse relationship between percentage absorption and the total amount of iron stores (gut mucosal cells have a regulatory rôle)
(iv) In health, 10% of dietary iron is absorbed—can increase to 30% in iron deficiency

3. Transport
Principally attached to the protein transferrin (a ß globulin).

4. Utilisation
Incorporation into haemoglobin, myoglobin and tissue enzymes (cytochromes, catalase and peroxidase).

5. Storage
Tissue iron stores (mainly in liver, bone marrow, spleen and muscle) normally amount to about 1 g:
(i) Ferritin—protein (apoferritin) shell surrounding a crystalline core of hydrated ferric oxide-phosphate. Iron can be readily mobilised from this molecule and made available for erythropoiesis
(ii) Haemosiderin—a macro-molecule, at least partly an

aggregation of ferritin molecules. The chief storage form, from which iron is less quickly mobilised
Normally two-thirds of storage iron is in the form of ferritin and one-third haemosiderin.
  Haemosiderin is increased in iron overload states.

6. *Requirements for iron balance*
(i) Vary considerably from infancy to puberty—from 0.3 mg/day to at least 1 mg/day
(ii) Adult males need 0.5–1.5 mg/day to compensate for losses (cell desquamation, sweat, urine)
(iii) Adult females need 1.0–3.0 mg/day to compensate for losses including (normal) menses and increased demand in pregnancy

Causes of deficiency
Iron imbalance occurs when requirements outstrip the availability of iron because of:
1. Inadequate dietary intake
2. Failure of absorption of dietary iron
3. Excessive iron loss—in particular blood loss
4. Increased utilisation—pregnancy

Pathogenesis
As the availability of iron stores becomes critical, erythropoiesis becomes abnormal and this results in:
1. Reduction in red cell size
2. Reduction in the concentration of haemoglobin in red cells
3. Fall in haemoglobin level and packed cell volume
With established iron deficiency, tissue changes may occur, notably in the gastrointestinal tract

Haematology
1. Anaemia, typically microcytic and hypochromic (Hb, MCV, MCH and MCHC decreased)
2. Blood film—hypochromia and microcytosis, variable anisocytosis, anisochromia and poikilocytosis
3. Bone marrow—absent iron stores

Biochemistry
1. Decreased serum iron
2. Increased total iron binding capacity (TIBC)—not invariable; TIBC may be normal or reduced in patients who also have infections or inflammatory/malignant diseases (see Fig. 2.1, p.6)
3. Decreased serum ferritin—levels generally reflect the mobilisable iron stores but values may be falsely raised as 'acute phase reactant' e.g. during infections, in active arthritis and in malignant disease

Clinical features
1. The commonest anaemia—may occur at any age but infants, women of reproductive age and the old are particularly at risk
2. Non-specific symptoms of anaemia—lethargy, dyspnoea on exertion, etc.
3. Symptoms of cardiovascular insufficiency, aggravated by anaemia—e.g. angina in patients with co-existing atherosclerosis
4. Features secondary to tissue changes:
   (i) Angular stomatitis
   (ii) Atrophic glossitis (pale, smooth tongue)
   (iii) Thinning and ridging of nails which break easily
   (iv) Koilonychia (spoon-shaped nails)
   (v) Post-cricoid web causing dysphagia (Brown–Kelly–Paterson or Plummer–Vinson syndrome)
   (vi) Atrophy of gastric mucosa
   (vii) Pruritus
   (viii) Pica

Associations
1. During growth:
   (i) At 6–24 months, due to diminished iron stores (especially in premature infants) and inadequate dietary intake
   (ii) At growth spurts—especially puberty
2. In pregnancy, particularly if dietary intake is poor
3. Dietary inadequacy, e.g. in vegans, low-income groups and the uninterested
4. Blood loss—common sites are:
   (i) Female genital tract (menorrhagia)
   (ii) Gastrointestinal tract, due to:
       a. Drugs – aspirin, NSAIDS, alcohol
       b. Hiatus hernia
       c. Peptic ulcer
       d. Carcinoma
       e. Haemorrhoids
       f. Colitis
       g. Hookworm
       h. Vascular lesions—hereditary haemorragic telangiectasia (Osler–Rendu–Weber syndrome), angiodysplasia
5. Malabsorption – e.g. post gastric surgery, coeliac disease

Treatment
1. Correction of underlying cause if possible, e.g.:
   (i) Low dietary intake—expert dietary guidance; continuing supplementation with iron for those adhering to a strict vegan diet for religious reasons
   (ii) Persisting excessive uterine blood loss—e.g. surgery for fibroids, oral contraceptive pill

    (iii) Gastrointestinal blood loss—withdrawal of irritant drugs; treatment of ulcerating lesions—surgical, H_2-blockers and proton-pump inhibitors

    (iv) Malabsorption—institution of gluten-free diet in coeliac disease. The post-gastrectomy patient may require a daily iron supplement for life

2. Replacement of depleted iron (blood transfusion is *rarely* indicated):

    (i) Oral iron—to provide at least 100 g elemental iron/day, e.g. ferrous sulphate 200 mg b.d. or t.d.s.
    Side-effects include nausea, abdominal pain and diarrhoea/constipation, often dose related

    (ii) Parenteral iron—very rarely necessary but sometimes required in severe malabsorption or where there is poor compliance or intolerance to oral iron. A significant proportion of the iron forms a non-utilisable complex
    Side-effects include pain and staining at the site of i.m. injection, and hypersensitivity reactions which can be severe

3. Assessment of response—in uncomplicated iron deficiency:

    (i) Haemoglobin rises by 0.1–0.2 g/dl/day
    (ii) Reticulocyte response relates to the degree of anaemia (but not as good an indicator as in treated pernicious anaemia)

4. Failure to respond may be due to:

    (i) Patient's failure to take the tablets
    (ii) Continuing iron loss (bleeding)
    (iii) Malabsorption
    (iv) Other diagnoses—thalassaemia trait, sideroblastic anaemia

5. Duration of therapy:

    (i) For 6–9 months—to replete marrow iron stores, assuming the original cause of iron deficiency is eliminated
    (ii) Prolonged indefinitely—in patients with frequent abnormal blood losses (e.g. menorrhagia) and those with continuing poor intake and/or malabsorption (e.g. post-gastrectomy syndrome)

2. Non-siferopenic hypochromic anaemias

Basic features
1. Red cell indices and blood film appearances *suggest* iron deficiency, although peripheral blood changes are not usually as marked as in moderate or severe iron deficiency
2. Erythropoiesis is abnormal because of ineffective iron utilisation with poor haemoglobinisation of red cell precursors
3. Bone marrow iron stores are normal or increased and sideroblasts may be frequent and abnormal

Causes
1. Secondary anaemias (see p.45):
   (i) Chronic infection/inflammation
   (ii) Malignancy
2. Thalassaemia (p.27)
3. Sideroblastic anaemia

Differentiation from iron deficiency (see Fig. 2.1)
The serum iron and total iron binding capacity (transferrin) are helpful but not diagnostic; it is quite possible to have co-existing ineffective iron utilisation *and* iron deficiency, as determined by bone marrow iron status, e.g. in rheumatoid arthritis.

SIDEROBLASTIC ANAEMIA

Classification
Not a single disease entity or a homogeneous group, but linked by definition—the presence of the ring sideroblast.
   There are three main categories:
1. Hereditary (sex-linked, ? other)
2. Primary acquired (sub-group of myelodysplastic disorders)
3. Secondary acquired (or 'associated'). Important associations are:
   (i) Drugs, e.g. antituberculous, notably isoniazid and pyrazinamide
   (ii) Poisons, e.g. lead, alcohol
   (iii) Nutritional deficiencies, especially in malabsorption states

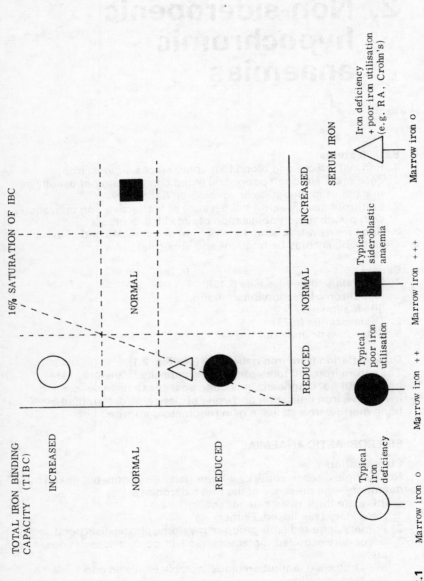

Fig. 2.1

(iv) A variety of haematological diseases, e.g. myeloproliferative diseases and leukaemias
(v) Chronic disorders—rheumatoid arthritis, carcinomatosis, uraemia, myxoedema

Pathogenesis
The crucial defect, or defects, is not delineated but abnormal deposition of iron in relation to erythroblast mitochondria is associated with:
1. Evidence of defective haem synthesis—increased free protoporphyrin is usual in the primary acquired form (see p.166)
2. Impaired synthesis of haemoglobin (with no evidence of a primary defect in globin synthesis)
3. Impaired iron utilisation and development of iron overload, severe in repeatedly transfused patients
4. Ineffective erythropoiesis, often with relative folate deficiency

Haematology
1. Anaemia:
   (i) Hereditary form—hypochromic, microcytic
   (ii) Acquired forms—normochromic or hypochromic, MCV normal or increased
2. Leucopenia and/or thrombocytopenia occur but there is no uniform pattern
3. Blood film—'dimorphic' pattern (due to the presence of two red cell populations) ± dysplastic features
4. Bone marrow—abundant iron stores and presence of diagnostic ring sideroblasts (≥6 iron granules arranged round the nucleus – see p.166)
5. Features of associated disease, e.g. leukaemia, myeloproliferative disease

Clinical features
1. Presentation:
   (i) Hereditary form—in childhood or early adult life
   (ii) Acquired form (primary)—usually in middle or old age
2. A long history of iron therapy with poor response is common
3. Anaemia—variable, from very mild to severe
4. Hepatomegaly and splenomegaly—common (overall)
5. Features of associated disease in secondary acquired form—e.g. malabsorption, leukaemia, alcoholism

Complications
1. Progressive iron overload, in those requiring repeated blood transfusions, leading to haemosiderosis
2. Development of frank malignancy, e.g. leukaemia

Treatment
1. Removal of associated pathology where possible, e.g. by withdrawal of alcohol
2. 'Trial by therapy', ideally in sequence, with assessment of response to each agent. Patients who respond to pyridoxine may do so slowly, over several months:
   (i)   Folic acid 5 mg daily (over half the patients are folate-depleted and some may be frankly megaloblastic)
   (ii) Pyridoxine hydrochloride (vitamin B_6)—at least 500 mg daily
   (iii) Other vitamins, e.g. ascorbic acid and riboflavin, may be given in addition to the above (of dubious value)
   (iv) Chelation of iron with desferrioxamine may delay the development of haemosiderosis—important in young patients
3. Avoidance of blood transfusions until absolutely necessary

Course and prognosis
Sideroblastic anaemias are often described as 'responsive' or 'non-responsive', in terms of increase in Hb level, to pharmacological doses of vitamin B_6.
1. Hereditary—80% are 'responsive', though the haematology does not revert completely to normal
2. Primary acquired—40% are 'responsive', but the response may be slight and is usually suboptimal
3. Secondary—60% are 'responsive', the response also depending on the effectiveness of the treatment of associated conditions
Severe refractory sideroblastic anaemias requiring regular transfusions and/or leukaemic transformation (5–10% cases) (see p.119) significantly reduce life expectancy.

3. Megaloblastic anaemias

DUE TO VITAMIN B_{12} DEFICIENCY

Basic nutritional features and metabolism of B_{12}

1. Dietary vitamin B_{12}
(i)   Only present in food of animal origin—important sources are red meats and dairy produce (B_{12} synthesised in the gut is not absorbed in man)
(ii) Cooking does not usually destroy vitamin B_{12}
(iii) Daily minimum requirement is $1-2\,\mu g$

2. Absorption
(i)   Vitamin B_{12} is liberated from foodstuffs in the stomach
(ii) Bound by intrinsic factor (a glycoprotein synthesised by the parietal cells) at an acid pH
(iii) Absorbed through the terminal ileal mucosa

3. Transport
(i)   Chiefly by transcobalamin II (a ß globulin)—rapid transport mechanism
(ii) To a lesser extent by transcobalamin I and III—though *most* vitamin B_{12} in serum is bound to transcobalamin I (an α globulin) which acts as a circulating reserve store of vitamin B_{12}

4. Metabolism
Vitamin B_{12} is essential for two reactions:
(i)   Isomerisation of methyl-malonyl CoA to succinyl CoA (a step in proprionic acid metabolism)
(ii) Conversion of homocysteine to methionine (by 5-methyl tetrahydrofolate transferase, which contains vitamin B_{12}) – the important defect, as formate derived from methionine and tetrahydrofolate are both crucial in folate metabolism and nucleic acid synthesis

5. Storage
Primarily hepatic (about 1.5 mg).
   Overall 2–3 mg, the requirement for 3–4 years if other sources unavailable

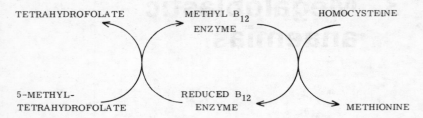

TETRAHYDROFOLATE   METHYL B_{12} HOMOCYSTEINE
                          ENZYME

5-METHYL-   REDUCED B_{12}
TETRAHYDROFOLATE   ENZYME   METHIONINE

Fig. 3.1 Vitamin B_{12} and folate relationship (in which the active co-enzyme form of folate is generated)

ADDISONIAN PERNICIOUS ANAEMIA (PA)

Pathogenesis
1. Development of gastric atrophy (associated with production of antibodies to parietal cells and intrinsic factor)
2. Failure of intrinsic factor production
3. Slow development of negative vitamin B_{12} balance and depletion of stores
4. Impaired nucleic acid synthesis due to lack of vitamin B_{12}
5. Nuclear maturation defect in cells with high growth rates, notably erythroblasts
6. Megaloblastic erythropoiesis
7. Neurological damage

Haematology
1. Anaemia, macrocytic (MCV increased, often >120 fl)
2. Moderate leucopenia due to neutropenia may occur
3. Platelets may be reduced
4. Blood film—oval macrocytes, anisocytosis and poikilocytosis; hypersegmented polymorphs (>5 nuclear lobes) often large forms—'macropolycytes'. Occasionally leucoerythroblastic film
5. Bone marrow—megaloblastic:
   (i)   Cellularity increased (erythroid hyperplasia)
   (ii) Erythroid nuclear/cytoplasmic asynchrony—primitive, large nuclei with open ('stippled') chromatin pattern, despite cytoplasmic maturation and haemoglobinisation
   (iii) Giant metamyelocytes
   (iv) Atypical megakaryocytes with hypersegmented nuclei (hyperpolyploidy)
6. Serum B_{12} level low, usually well below 160 ng/l (but important to know the normal range for the assay used, microbiological or radioisotopic dilution)

Biochemistry
1. Increased unconjugated bilirubin, reflecting mild haemolysis and ineffective erythropoiesis (also in folate deficiency)
2. Increased serum lactic dehydrogenase (LDH), reflecting ineffective, megaloblastic erythropoiesis (also in folate deficiency)
3. Increased excretion of methyl-malonic acid in urine (with valine load) due to lack of B_{12} co-enzyme

Immunology
1. Parietal cell antibodies in serum (80%+ of patients, but not specific)
2. Intrinsic factor (IF) antibodies (more specific)
   Type I 'blocking' antibodies in 55% of patients
   Type II 'binding' antibodies in 35% of patients

Other investigations
1. Schilling test—malabsorption of B_{12} corrected by addition of intrinsic factor (one version is the differential absorption and excretion of B_{12} with and without intrinsic factor, using ^{57}Co- and ^{58}Co-labelled B_{12})
2. Gastric biopsy—proximal two-thirds of stomach atrophic (biopsies rarely done)
3. Deoxyuridine suppression test (incorporation of ^{3}H-thymidine into the DNA of marrow cells suppressed by pre-incubation with deoxyuridine)—subnormal suppression (also in folate deficiency) correctable by B_{12} or folinic acid

Clinical features
1. The majority of patients are middle-aged or elderly
2. Greater incidence in related people than in the general population, though exact genetic basis not clear, and in patients with blood group A, HLA-A_3
3. An insidious onset is usual
4. Anaemia—may be severe and precipitate cardiac decompensation
   Note: B_{12} deficiency is not invariably associated with anaemia
5. Mild jaundice is sometimes detectable
6. Glossitis—soreness with no visible changes may progress to red tongue with marked loss of papillae
7. Neurological features:
   (i)   Paraesthesiae in hands and feet (early peripheral neuropathy)
   (ii) Established peripheral neuropathy with 'glove and stocking' sensory loss and motor weakness

(iii) Involvement of dorsal and lateral columns of spinal cord (often patchy lesions)—loss of proprioception and vibration sense ± motor signs

(iv) Combined effect of peripheral and central changes — typically, diminished reflexes, extensor plantar responses and sensory losses—sub-acute combined degeneration (SACD)

(v) Mental changes, from mild memory loss to psychosis

(vi) Optic atrophy

8. Associated autoimmune disorders—myxoedema, hypoparathyroidism, Addison's disease, diabetes, hypogammaglobulinaemia—may occur

Treatment

Neurological damage can be precipitated by treating incorrectly with folic acid.

1. Initial treatment is often given as the $1000\,\mu g$ B_{12} flushing dose in the Schilling test

2. In the presence of neurological damage—weekly B_{12} ($500-1000\,\mu g$ hydroxocobalamin) initially, though rationale for 'intensive' therapy is obscure

3. Maintenance—$1000\,\mu g$ hydroxocobalamin every 3 months is usually adequate

Other causes of vitamin B_{12} deficiency

1. Dietary deficiency—in very poor socioeconomic groups and in strict vegetarians (vegans)

2. Post gastric surgery:
   (i) Total gastrectomy—when B_{12} stores are exhausted, usually after several years
   (ii) Partial gastrectomy—possibly related to secondary atrophic gastritis
       Note: B_{12} deficiency is much less common than iron deficiency

3. Non-Addisonian 'pernicious anaemia':
   (i) In association with hypogammaglobulinaemia—gastric atrophy, achlorhydria and absent intrinsic factor but *no* antibodies and a younger age group than Addisonian PA
   (ii) In infancy—selective failure of intrinsic factor, normal mucosa
   (iii) Juvenile PA—failure of intrinsic factor secretion with gastric atrophy (rarely, with antibodies)
   (iv) Congenital transcobalamin II deficiency
   (v) Congenital methyl-malonic aciduria

4. Small intestinal 'sequestration':
   (i) The 'blind-loop' syndrome—in association with strictures, anastomoses or diverticula. The anatomical abnormalities

encourage abnormal gut flora which compete for available vitamin B_{12}

(ii) Infestation with fish tapeworm (*Diphyllobothrium latum*), which is avid for vitamin B_{12}

5. Selective malabsorption, with proteinuria (Imerslund–Gräsbeck syndrome) (rare). Absorption may be reversibly defective in severe B_{12}/folate deficiency states

6. Post-resection of terminal ileum, e.g. for Crohn's disease

7. Tropical sprue

8. Prolonged nitrous oxide anaesthesia

DUE TO FOLATE DEFICIENCY

Basic nutritional features and metabolism of folate

1. Dietary folate

(i) Important sources are liver, kidney and fresh green leafy vegetables

(ii) 'Folate' is a term covering a family of compounds

(iii) Natural polyglutamates differ in the number of glutamyl residues (chief forms are tri- and hepta-glutamates)

(iv) Cooking destroys at least half the folate in food (50–90%)

(v) Requirements are difficult to assess as calculations have been in terms of synthetic folate (minimum recommended: 100–200 µg daily)

(vi) The level of daily dietary intake at which megaloblastic change develops is about 30 µg

2. Absorption

(i) Synthetic folic acid (pteroylglutamic acid) is absorbed in the jejunum by an active transport mechanism

(ii) Food folates require deconjugation by intestinal conjugase

(iii) Absorption of all forms is chiefly in the jejunum

3. Metabolism

(i) Reduced, formylated and methylated forms result from metabolism during absorption and in the liver

(ii) Folates in the plasma are probably protein-bound but are rapidly taken up by the tissues

(iii) Tetrahydrofolate is essential in thymidylate and hence DNA synthesis

4. Storage

(i) Mainly hepatic, 6–10 mg

(ii) The stores represent the normal requirements for 3–4 months

(iii) There can be quite rapid depletion in situations where body requirements are increased.

Causes of deficiency
Nutritional imbalance is much more frequent than in the case of
vitamin B$_{12}$ and there are many situations which can result in frank
deficiency and anaemia. Negative folate balance may result from:
1. Inadequate intake
2. Malabsorption
3. Increased utilisation
4. Interference with metabolism by drugs
5. Various combinations of 1–4

Pathogenesis
1. Impairment of nucleic acid synthesis as in vitamin B$_{12}$
   deficiency
2. Nuclear maturation defect
3. Megaloblastic erythropoiesis

Haematology
1. Essentially as in vitamin B$_{12}$ deficiency
2. Howell–Jolly bodies and target cells in the blood film would
   suggest splenic atrophy (coeliac disease)
3. Bone marrow—the classical megaloblastic changes may be
   masked, or partially so in:
   (i) Iron deficiency (co-existent)
   (ii) Poor iron utilisation states, e.g. inflammatory diseases and
        malignancy
   Masked, mild or 'intermediate' megaloblastosis is frequent in
   the folate depletion which occurs in a wide range of conditions
4. Reduced folate levels—serum levels are labile and red cell levels
   are a better reflection of tissue folate

Assay
1. Microbiological—e.g. using *Lactobacillus casei*, the growth of
   which depends on availability of folate
2. Radioisotopic dilution—now reliable and, unlike microbiological
   techniques, not interfered with by antibiotics or folate
   antagonists (e.g. methotrexate)

Clinical features
1. May occur at any age
2. Degrees of folate deficiency are very common and mild
   deficiency states are frequently unrecognised
3. The clinical picture is multivarious because of the variety of
   possible underlying causes
4. The onset may be insidious or rapid, as when negative folate
   balance is precipitated by, e.g. infection
5. Anaemia and sometimes slight jaundice
6. Glossitis
7. No defined neurological changes; any cerebral effects uncertain

Associations

1. Dietary inadequacy
(i)   Old people living alone (on 'tea and biscuits')
(ii) Subjects on reducing, 'fad' or gastric diets
(iii) Vegans (though diet often adequate for folate)
(iv) Pregnancy (late) when folate requirements increase
(v)   Infancy—chiefly in poor socioeconomic groups
(vi) Intensive care patients on prolonged i.v. fluid regimens

2. Malabsorption
(i)   Coeliac disease, severe or subclinical
(ii) Enteropathies associated with dermatitis herpetiformis or lymphoma
(iii) Tropical sprue (especially in the Far East and Caribbean)

3. Diseases/situations with increased folate requirements
(i)   Haemolytic anaemias and anaemias associated with ineffective erythropoiesis (e.g. thalassaemia)
(ii)   Myeloproliferative diseases, e.g. myelofibrosis
(iii) Malignancy
(iv)   Pregnancy
(v)   Infections with florid cellular reaction
(vi)   Inflammatory diseases, e.g. rheumatoid arthritis, Crohn's disease
(vii) Exfoliative skin disease
(viii) Chronic renal dialysis

4. Ingestion of anti-folate drugs
(i)   Anticonvulsants (e.g. phenytoin)—interfere with the metabolism of folate (possibly, crucially, in the liver)
(ii) Alcohol—interferes with folate utilisation (as well as directly damaging cells)
      Note: Alcoholics may also have folate deficient diets
(iii) Various—nitrofurantoin, dapsone, salazopyrine, oral contraceptive pill

Treatment
1. The treatment of folate deficiency without having established the cause may delay a definitive diagnosis
2. Folic acid therapy is contraindicated if there is *any* suspicion of B$_{12}$ deficiency (neurological changes may be precipitated)
3. Routinely, folic acid 5 mg daily is more than adequate

FURTHER ADVANCED READING

Chanarin I 1990 The megaloblastic anaemias, 3rd edn. Blackwell, Oxford

4. Haemolytic anaemias

There are two broad categories:
A. Hereditary
B. Acquired

Basic features
1. Abnormal and accelerated destruction of red cells and, in some anaemias, their precursors
2. Increased breakdown of haemoglobin which may result in:
   (i) Increased bilirubin level (mainly indirect-reacting) with jaundice
   (ii) Increased faecal and urinary urobilinogen
   (iii) Haemoglobinaemia, methaemalbuminaemia, haemoglobinuria and haemosiderinuria (where there is significant intravascular haemolysis)
3. Bone marrow compensatory reaction:
   (i) Erythroid hyperplasia with accelerated production of red cells, reflected by reticulocytosis and slight macrocytosis in peripheral blood
   (ii) Expansion of bone marrow in infants and children with severe chronic haemolysis—changes in bone configuration, visible on X-ray
4. The balance between red cell destruction and marrow compensation determines the severity of anaemia

A. HEREDITARY HAEMOLYTIC ANAEMIAS*

HEREDITARY SPHEROCYTOSIS (HS)

Genetics
1. Inherited as autosomal dominant but the severity of anaemia and degree of spherocytosis may not be uniform within an affected family
2. Commonest in people of northern European stock

---

*To include haemoglobinopathies and the thalassaemias, where other mechanisms contribute to the haematological abnormalities

Pathogenesis
The fundamental abnormality is probably in spectrin, the contractile protein of the red cell membrane.

Sequelae
1. Sequestration of red cells in the spleen (due to reduced erythrocyte deformability)
2. Depletion of membrane lipid
3. Loss of cell surface area relative to volume
4. Tendency to spherocytosis
5. Influx and efflux of sodium increased
6. Rapid ATP utilisation and increased glycolysis
7. Premature red cell destruction

Haematology
1. Anaemia—mild in compensated cases; MCV usually normal; MCHC may be increased
2. Reticulocytosis
3. Blood film—red cells appear spherocytic and some are small ('microspherocytes')
4. Coombs test negative
5. Increased red cell osmotic fragility (spherocytes lyse in *higher* concentrations of saline than normal red cells)
6. Survival of ^{51}Cr labelled cells reduced, with increased splenic sequestration
7. Increased autohaemolysis

Biochemistry
Raised bilirubin (mainly indirect-reacting).
   Note: obstructive jaundice, with increased direct-reacting bilirubin, may develop due to gall-stones, a consequence of increased pigment excretion.

Clinical features
1. The majority of patients present before puberty
2. The diagnosis is sometimes made much later in life, and by chance
3. Anaemia and jaundice—the severity depending on the rate of haemolysis and degree of compensation
4. Splenomegaly

Complications
1. 'Haemolytic crisis', with more pronounced jaundice due to accelerated haemolysis (may be precipitated by infection)
2. 'Aplastic crisis' with dramatic fall in haemoglobin level (and reticulocyte count)—decompensation, usually due to maturation arrest and often associated with megaloblastic change; may be precipitated by infection, notably with parvovirus

3. Folate deficiency caused by increased bone marrow requirement
4. Pigment gall-stones, in approximately half of untreated patients
5. Leg ulcers

Treatment
1. Definitive—splenectomy, for moderate to severe cases.
   Therapeutic gain:
   (i)   Although spherocytosis persists, red cell life span becomes
         essentially normal and complications are thereby
         prevented
   (ii) Should be carried out early in severe cases but not before 5
         years of age
   Pneumococcal vaccine should be given pre-splenectomy and
   penicillin V 250 mg b.d. subsequently, indefinitely, as prophylaxis
   against potentially fatal infections, e.g. pneumococcal
2. Supportive:
   (i)   Folic acid supplement
   (ii) Blood transfusion for crises

HEREDITARY ELLIPTOCYTOSIS

1. Genetics—autosomal dominant
2. Pathogenesis—predominantly a spectrin defect
3. Haematology:
   (i)   Anaemia—mild to moderate
   (ii) Blood film—oval red cells; pyropoikilocytosis in rare
         homozygous form
   (iii) Spleen rarely enlarged
   (iv) Osmotic fragility—normal or slightly increased
4. Treatment:
   Mild cases—observation
   More severe cases—as for hereditary spherocytosis

CONGENITAL HAEMOLYTIC ANAEMIAS DUE TO ENZYME DEFECTS

GLUCOSE-6-PHOSPHATE DEHYDROGENASE (G-6-PD) DEFICIENCY

G-6-PD is the first enzyme in the pentose phosphate pathway of
glucose metabolism. (see Fig. 4.1). Deficiency diminishes the
reductive energy of the red cell and may result in haemolysis, the
severity of which depends on the quantity and type of G-6-PD and
the nature of the haemolytic agent (usually an oxidation-reduction
mediator).

Genetics
1. Transmitted as sex-linked recessive by a gene located on the X-
   chromosome (like haemophilia)
2. Disease fully expressed in hemizygous male and homozygous
   female

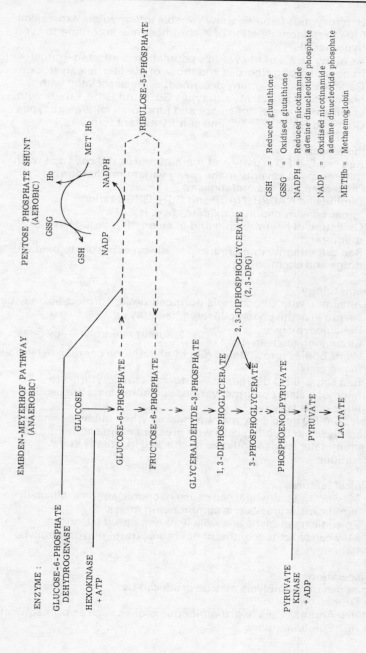

Fig. 4.1 Glycolytic pathways in the red cell

3. Heterozygous females show variable intermediate expression (due to random deletion of X-chromosome, according to Lyon hypothesis)
4. As many as 3% of the world's population is affected—most frequent among Negroes and those of Mediterranean stock.
5. Genetic variants—many described; some associated with normal enzyme activity e.g. types Gd^{A+} and Gd^{B+}, others with varying degrees of deficiency and functional failure e.g. types Gd^{A-} and $Gd^{Mediterranean}$ and sundry mutant forms

Pathogenesis
1. Red cell G-6-PD activity and prematurely as red cells age (with differences in severity in the many variant/mutant forms)
2. Decreased glucose metabolism
3. Diminished NADPH: NADP and GSH: GSSG ratios
4. Impaired elimination of oxidants (e.g. H_2O_2)
5. Oxidation of haemoglobin and of sulphydryl groups in the membrane
6. Red cell integrity impaired, especially on exposure to oxidant drugs and chemicals

Haematology
1. Anaemia, when it occurs, is normochromic, normocytic; may be severe in acute uncompensated haemolysis
2. Reticulocytosis ⎫
3. Circulating nucleated red cells ⎬ during haemolytic episodes
4. Heinz bodies (precipitated globin-glutathione complexes) visible in red cells
5. Red cell G-6-PD decreased—a direct assay (erythrocyte haemolysates) confirms. Various screening tests are used in large-scale surveys
Note: G-6-PD deficiency may be masked when older cells have haemolysed and young cells with greater enzyme content predominate; levels should be re-checked in 'steady state' conditions

Clinical features
1. May occur at any age; can cause neonatal jaundice; clinically significant expression is commoner in males
2. Episodic haemolytic anaemia with non-specific features
3. May cause acute (common) or chronic (rare) non-spherocytic haemolysis

Associations
Episodes of haemolysis may be produced by:
1. Drugs:
    (i)   Antimalarials (e.g. 8-aminoquinolones such as primaquine)
    (ii) Sulphonamides

(iii) Nitrofurans, e.g. nitrofurantoin (Furadantin)
(iv) Dapsone (as used in leprosy)
(v) Doxorubicin
2. The fava bean (broad bean, *Vicia fava*)—on ingestion or exposure to pollen from the bean's flower (hence 'favism')
3. Infection (in the more susceptible subjects)

Treatment
1. Discontinue exposure to offending drug or other agent
2. Transfusions, rarely needed
3. Folic acid (in acute haemolytic episodes)

PYRUVATE KINASE (PK) DEFICIENCY

Pyruvate kinase is an enzyme active in the penultimate conversion in the Embden–Meyerhof pathway. Deficiency is rare but can cause moderately severe haemolytic anaemia (*not* drug-induced).

Genetics
1. Transmitted as autosomal recessive—significant haemolysis is seen in homozygotes
2. Found predominantly in people of northern European stock and much less common than G-6-PD deficiency in the world population
3. Deficiency is not simply quantitative and probably often reflects the production of PK variants with abnormal characteristics

Pathogenesis
1. Defective red cell glycolysis with reduced ATP formation
2. Red cells become rigid, deformed and metabolically and physically vulnerable (reticulocytes are less vulnerable because of their ability to generate ATP by oxidative phosphorylation)

Haematology
1. Features of haemolysis with relatively marked reticulocytosis and many poikilocytes, 'prickle cells' and distorted cells (spherocytes are uncommon)
2. Erythrocyte PK activity is decreased, to 5–20% of normal; 2,3,DPG and other glycolytic intermediate metabolites are increased
3. Autohaemolysis is decreased by ATP (*not* glucose as in HS)

Clinical features
1. Usually presents in early life (sometimes as jaundice in the newborn)
2. Variable severity

3. Splenomegaly is common but not invariable
4. Late—pigment gall-stones, haemosiderosis (from multiple transfusions)

Treatment
1. Transfusions as required
2. Splenectomy (if transfusion requirements increase)
3. Folic acid

Other enzyme deficiencies have been reported—they are very rare and outside the scope of this book

THE HAEMOGLOBINOPATHIES

Definition
Genetically-determined abnormalities in the molecular structure of the globin chains of haemoglobin
   While a vast number of abnormal haemoglobins have now been described, the majority are of no clinical consequence.

HAEMOGLOBIN S

Genetics
1. Transmitted as incomplete autosomal dominant
2. Homozygotes (two abnormal genes) synthesise no HbA and their red cells contain 90–100% HbS
3. Heterozygotes (one abnormal gene) have red cells which contain 20–40% HbS
4. Largely found in Negro populations—the highest carrier rate is in central Africa (20%)

Basic defect and pathology
A single amino-acid substitution (valine for glutamic acid) in the β polypeptide chain. This simple alteration has the following consequences:
1. HbS has a higher net electrical charge than HbA—hence a different electrophoretic mobility
2. HbS in the reduced form (deoxygenated) is less soluble than HbA and the molecules form rod-like 'tactoids'—these in turn distort the red cell, which takes on the sickle form
3. Sickle cells are prematurely destroyed, causing a haemolytic anaemia
4. Sickle cells result in increased blood viscosity with impaired blood flow and initiate thrombi

SICKLE CELL ANAEMIA
Homozygous, SS disease

Haematology
1. Anaemia, moderate to severe normochromic, normocytic
2. Reticulocytosis
3. Neutrophilia is common
4. Platelets—often increased
5. Blood film—sickle cells, increased polychromasia, nucleated red cells and target cells (Howell–Jolly bodies may indicate hyposplenism)
6. ESR—low (sickle cells fail to form rouleaux)
7. Hb electrophoresis—HbS migrates slower than HbA, giving the diagnostic SS pattern (see Fig. 4.2)

Biochemistry
Features reflecting haemolysis.

Clinical features
1. Usually manifest in infancy
2. Signs of physical underdevelopment often become apparent
3. Symptoms and signs reflecting haemolytic anaemia
4. Symptoms and signs relating to thrombotic phenomena
    (i) Abdominal pain, e.g. due to splenic infarction, gallstones
    (ii) Chest pain
    (iii) Bone pain—at any site, but specifically in dactylitis (hand/foot syndrome) and aseptic necrosis of femoral heads
    (iv) Haematuria
    (v) Priapism
    (vi) A variety of neurological changes—coma, fits, CVAs
5. Splenomegaly—in young children. Recurrent infarcts result in decreasing spleen size and ultimately 'autosplenectomy' in some patients
6. Leg ulcers

Crises
1. Infarctive—episodes, usually painful, as listed above, precipitated by reduced pO_2, vascular stasis (as in circulatory failure and dehydration), reduced blood pH
2. 'Aplastic'—failure of marrow compensation, often precipitated by infection, notably with parvovirus. Folate deficiency may be an underlying factor
3. Haemolytic—accelerated haemolysis may occur, e.g. during infections but severe episodes usually reflect co-existing G-6-PD deficiency (see p.20)
4. Sequestration—rapidly enlarging spleen and liver; seen in young children

Treatment/management
1. Of the steady state:
    (i) Adequate prophylaxis against, and treatment of, infection

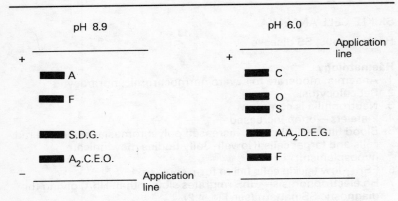

Citrate agar gel electrophoresis (pH 6.0) separates HbS and D, C and E —not distinguishable by cellulose acetate electrophoresis (pH 8.9)

Fig. 4.2A Hb electrophoresis at alkaline and acid pH

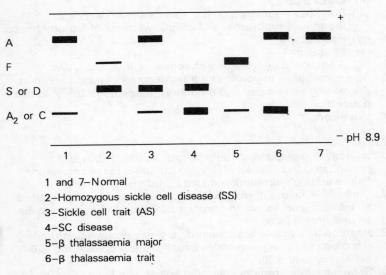

1 and 7—Normal
2—Homozygous sickle cell disease (SS)
3—Sickle cell trait (AS)
4—SC disease
5—β thalassaemia major
6—β thalassaemia trait

Fig. 4.2B Electrophoretic patterns for common haemoglobinopathies and thalassaemias

(ii) Avoidance of situations which precipitate infarction, e.g. hypoxia, as in air travel

(iii) Folic acid—daily supplement

2. Of crises:
   (i) Correction of precipitating factors—re-hydration, treatment of infection
   (ii) Transfusion—exchange in deteriorating situations; additive in less severe cases
   (iii) Anti-sickling drugs—an agent of proven value for general use has yet to be found

3. Genetic counselling and antenatal diagnosis

Course and prognosis

1. Death in infancy or childhood is usual in underdeveloped countries

2. Variation in survival data partly reflects standards of medical care. Milder forms compatible with long survival are now well recognised

SICKLE CELL TRAIT

Heterozygous (AS) form.

As HbS concentration in red cells is low, sickling does not occur under normal conditions.

Haematology

1. Indices are usually normal

2. Blood film—normal or mildly hypochromic with a few target cells

3. Sickle cell preparation—reducing agents (e.g. sodium metabisulphite) induce sickling in vitro

4. Hb electrophoresis—AS pattern (HbA ≈ 50%, HbS ≈ 50%)

Clinical features

1. Usually asymptomatic

2. Haematuria *may* occur

3. Infarctions are rare (but may occur during flights in unpressurised aircraft)

Significance

Genetic implications—counselling is indicated.

HAEMOGLOBIN C

Basic features and pathology

1. Carrier state 2% in Negroes (higher incidence in northern Ghana where the mutant presumably arose)

2. Amino-acid substitution (the same codon in the β chain as in HbS)—lysine for glutamic acid
3. HbC tends to form rhomboidal crystals with increases in osmolality—red cell deformability is impaired and splenic sequestration increased

HAEMOGLOBIN C DISEASE (Homozygous form, CC)

Haematology
1. Anaemia, usually mild, haemolytic
2. Blood film—numerous target cells and also small spherocytes (the result of membrane loss in the spleen)
3. Hb electrophoresis—CC pattern; slightly increased HbF

Clinical features
1. Less severe than HbSS
2. Splenomegaly
3. Dehydration may provoke marked haemolysis and cause microcirculatory problems

HAEMOGLOBIN C TRAIT (Heterozygous form, AC)

Asymptomatic, with only genetic significance.

HAEMOGLOBIN SC DISEASE

Combination of HbS and HbC.

Haematology
1. Anaemia, if present, is usually mild, haemolytic
2. Blood film—many target cells; sickle cells may be seen
3. Sickle cell preparations—positive
4. Hb electrophoresis—SC pattern (HbS ≈ 50%, HbC ≈ 50%)

Clinical features
Similar to, but less severe than, sickle cell anaemia. Severe infarctions may occur, e.g. during pregnancy or the puerperium, and prove fatal. Proliferative retinopathy more common than in SS.

HAEMOGLOBIN S/THAL

Combination of HbS and β thalassaemia trait. Haematology and clinical features vary—the severity depends upon the amount of normal adult haemoglobin synthesised (from 0–30%): with no HbA, the disease is comparable to sickle cell anaemia.

HAEMOGLOBIN D AND E

These β chain variants are not uncommon in a world context but cause relatively little morbidity.

OTHER HAEMOGLOBINOPATHIES (rare but of academic importance)

HAEMOGLOBIN M

Several M haemoglobin variants are known.

Basic features
Amino-acid substitutions result in the formation of stable complexes with iron—the net results are comparable to methaemoglobin formation (see p. 43). Present with familial cyanosis.

UNSTABLE HAEMOGLOBINS (e.g. Köln and Zurich)

Structural abnormalities in globin chains resulting in decreased stability of the haemoglobin molecule. Only seen in the heterozygous state.

Haematology
1. Haemolytic anaemia of variable severity
2. Blood film—Heinz bodies
3. Heat-labile haemoglobin demonstrable in vitro

HAEMOGLOBINS WITH ALTERED OXYGEN AFFINITY

1. Increased affinity—relative tissue hypoxia results in increased erythropoietin and hence erythrocytosis, e.g. Hb Yakima
2. Decreased affinity—converse effects with decreased stimulation of erythropoiesis, e.g. Hb Seattle

THE THALASSAEMIAS

Definition
Genetically determined defects in globin chain synthesis causing disordered haemoglobin production and abnormal erythropoiesis.

Basis features
1. The alpha (α) thalassaemias are seen particularly in peoples from the Chinese sub-continent, SE Asia and Africa; the beta (β) thalassaemias occur with highest frequency among those of Mediterranean and African origin, though with appreciable incidence in the Middle East and Asia. There is a selective

advantage for the thalassaemia heterozygote, in ameliorating the effects of malaria, which has influenced the geographical pattern of the disease.

In many populations α and β thalassaemia and structural haemoglobin variants (haemoglobinopathies) exist together, resulting in a wide spectrum of clinical disorders.

2. The degree of deficiency of globin chain synthesis in both the principal types of thalassaemia varies according to the nature of the genetic defects and whether heterozygous or homozygous. The clinical severity varies accordingly.
3. Decrease in α or β chain synthesis has a deleterious effect on red cell production with impaired haemoglobinisation.
4. There is unbalanced chain synthesis leading to a relative excess of one of the globin chains which may precipitate/aggregate and form intracellular inclusions, affecting erythroblast maturation, causing ineffective erythropoiesis and haemolysis, decreased membrane deformability and metabolic vulnerability.

β THALASSAEMIA—MAJOR, INTERMEDIA, 'HOMOZYGOUS'

Thalassaemia major refers to patients with severe β thalassaemia where regular blood transfusions are required. Both β globin genes (chromosome 11) are affected by a β thalassaemia mutation. Patients also 'homozygous' for β thalassaemia but with milder disease severity, e.g. not needing frequent, regular transfusions, are said to have thalassaemia intermedia. There is a spectrum of disease severity which relates to chain imbalance modified by the nature of the specific mutation(s), the capacity for α chain/HbF synthesis and the presence or absence of α thalassaemic mutations.

Pathogenesis
1. A double heterozygous state for two different mutations is usual rather than a strict homozygous state; large number of potential interactions of specific mutations possible
2. Variable suppression of β chain synthesis—complete (β°) or variably decreased (β^+); α chain excess
3. Variable degree of α chain activation and increase in fetal haemoglobin (HbF); modulates chain imbalance and improves red cell production (thereby *decreasing* clinical severity)
4. Coincidental inheritance of an α thalassaemia gene can also reduce the imbalance of chain synthesis
5. Increased but ineffective erythropoiesis with many red cell precursors prematurely destroyed—related to α chain excess
6. Shortened red cell life-span—variable splenic sequestration

Sequelae
1. Hyperplastic marrow—bone marrow expansion with cortical thinning
2. Increased iron absorption and iron overload (especially with repeated blood transfusions) resulting in:
   (i)   Cirrhosis of the liver
   (ii) Endocrine disturbances
3. Hypersplenism:
   (i)   Plasma volume expansion
   (ii)   Shortened red cell life (of autologous *and* donor cells)
   (iii) Leucopenia
   (iv)   Thrombocytopenia

Haematology
1. Anaemia—hypochromic, microcytic
2. Reticulocytosis
3. Leucopenia and thrombocytopenia may develop
4. Blood film—target cells and nucleated red cells
5. ^{51}Cr-labelled red cell life-span reduced (but the ineffective erythropoiesis is more important in the production of anaemia)
6. Haemoglobin F raised ('compensatory')
7. Bone marrow—hyperplastic and may be megaloblastic (due to folate depletion)

Biochemistry
1. Raised bilirubin (chiefly indirect-reacting)
2. Evidence of deranged liver function (late, as cirrhosis develops)
3. Evidence of endocrine abnormalities, e.g. diabetes (late)

Clinical features
1. Failure to thrive in early childhood is a common presentation
2. Anaemia
3. Jaundice, usually slight
4. Hepatosplenomegaly, which may be massive
5. Abnormal ('mongoloid') facies and fractures, due to marrow expansion and abnormal bone structure
6. Stunting due to chronic anaemia, protein lack and endocrine disturbances

Complications
Even in carefully managed patients, the following features may develop:
1. Endocrine disturbances, e.g. delayed puberty, diabetes, hypothyroidism, hypoparathyroidism, hypoadrenalism
2. Cirrhosis of the liver and liver failure
3. Cardiac failure due to anaemia, increased plasma volume and iron overload

Because of the variability in the severity of the fundamental defects there is a spectrum of clinical severity which considerably influences management and the full clinical 'syndrome' described applies to β thalassaemia major.

Treatment

Of severe forms
1. Hypertransfusion regimes (keeping Hb > 10 g/dl) suppresses ineffective endogenous haemopoiesis, with less growth and developmental retardation and fewer skeletal abnormalities
2. Iron chelation:
   (i) Desferrioxamine (25–50 mg/kg body weight) by subcutaneous infusion over 10–12 hours daily
        Side effects of desferrioxamine (ophthalmic (colour and night blindness) and auditory (high-tone hearing loss))
   (ii) Oral agents, e.g. L_1 (1,2 dimethyl-3-hydroxypyrid-4-one) will considerably delay development of iron overload and cirrhosis.
3. Splenectomy—reduces transfusion requirements if hypersplenism has developed
4. Folic acid supplements
5. Bone marrow transplantation—20% procedural mortality
6. Supportive care of patient and family; genetic counselling

Preventative
1. Genetic counselling
2. Antenatal diagnosis ± therapeutic abortion

Course and progress
In underdeveloped countries severely affected children usually die before puberty; with careful management such patients may survive much longer.

β THALASSAEMIA—HETEROZYGOUS FORMS (MINOR, TRAIT)

Pathogenesis
Typically, one β chain gene affected by a mutation decreasing or abolishing function (β^+ or β°) but genetic variants exist.

Haematology
1. Hb level usually normal or slightly reduced
2. RBC usually $> 5.5 \times 10^{12}$; MCV consistently low
3. Hypochromia, microcytosis and target cells in film
4. Hb A_2 increased (> 4%); may be lower if patient is iron-deficient; genetic variants with increased HbF and normal/low HbA_2 levels also occur

Clinical features
Often discovered following a routine blood test (low MCV)—usually asymptomatic.

α THALASSAEMIAS

More than 30 molecular mutations have been described—some abolish α gene expression (α°), others result in variably reduced expression (α⁺). There is considerable possible heterogeneity in the globin chain synthetic defect and clinical picture. However, there are basically four clinical syndromes of increasing severity in α thalassaemia due to inheritance of mutations affecting one, two, three or four of the α globin genes (chromosomes 16)—hydrops fetalis/Hb Barts syndrome, haemoglobin H disease, α thalassaemia trait and the 'silent carrier' state

HYDROPS FETALIS (Hb BARTS) SYNDROME

Pathogenesis
1. Homozygous state for α° results in failure to produce any α globin
2. Only Hb Barts (γ_4), HbH (β_4) produced—both functionally incompetent in terms of oxygen transport

Clinical features
The stillborn infants are grossly oedematous (hydrops fetalis) because of congestive heart failure due to severe anaemia.

HAEMOGLOBIN H (HbH) DISEASE

Pathogenesis
1. Single fully functional α globin gene; sometimes associated with elongated α globin chain production and resulting Hb Constant Spring which migrates slowly on electrophoresis
2. Excess β chain synthesis with production of HbH (β_4) which comprises 5–30% of the total haemoglobin; large amounts of Hb Barts are also produced at birth
3. HbH renders red cells vulnerable to oxidative stress, precipitates as the cells age and causes haemolysis

Haematology
1. Moderate reduction in Hb level (usually 7–10 g/dl)
2. Hypochromia, microcytosis and red cell fragmentation; 10–100% of red cells contain HbH 'golf-ball' inclusion bodies (demonstrated typically by cresyl blue incubation); reticulocytosis

Clinical features

Symptoms and signs of anaemia; splenomegaly; development of 'typical' thalassaemic features, e.g. facies unusual.

Treatment

1. Folic acid supplements
2. Avoidance of oxidant drugs
3. Prompt treatment of infection; occasionally transfusions may be required
4. Splenectomy only indicated if hypersplenism develops

α THALASSAEMIA MINOR OR TRAIT

Pathogenesis

Inactivation/deletion of both α globin genes on one chromosome or functional loss of one α gene on each chromosome 16.

Haematology

1. Essentially as for β thalassaemia trait except HbA_2 not increased
2. HbH inclusions may be detected in blood film occasionally

Diagnosis

Although Hb Barts is increased in the newborn there is no ready diagnostic marker of the disorder. Globin chain synthesis studies can be misleading and identification of gene abnormalities is not yet feasible as a routine investigation. In practice the diagnosis is usually based on:
1. Consistent haematological picture
2. Exclusion of iron deficiency (though this can co-exist)
3. Exclusion of β thalassaemia trait
4. Evidence of inheritance from family studies

Clinical features

As for β thalassaemia trait. Sometimes causes neonatal hyperbilirubinaemia. As in all the thalassaemia syndromes, it is important to investigate the families of patients to establish the type and severity of the defect. Genetic counselling may be indicated.

'SILENT CARRIER' FOR α THALASSAEMIA

Associated with the presence of three rather than four functional α globin genes. Impairment in α globin chain synthesis is very mild with virtually normal haematology apart from a slightly low MCV.

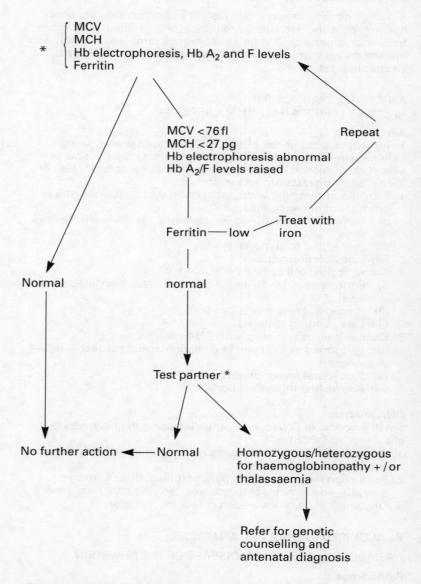

Fig. 4.3 Prenatal investigation of couples at risk for thalassaemia or haemoglobinopathies

HAEMOGLOBIN E DISEASE

A β chain gene mutation which results in a structurally abnormal haemoglobin and decreased production of β globin mRNA. High frequency in parts of SE Asia. Homozygous form is associated with marked microcytosis but only mild anaemia. Diagnosed by Hb electrophoresis.

ANTENATAL DIAGNOSIS IN HAEMOGLOBINOPATHIES/THALASSAEMIA

Aim

To identify couples at risk of having a child with severe haemo-globinopathy (SS, SC, SD, SE) or thalassaemia major in time to allow first or second trimester diagnosis and therapeutic abortion.
   The following tests can be performed:
1. Fetal blood sampling with globin chain synthesis—identifies products of mutant gene loci:
    (i)   Performed at 18–20 weeks gestation; results available in 10 days
    (ii) Procedural fetal mortality = 5%
    (iii) Late abortion required
2. Amniotic fluid cell culture with DNA analysis:
    (i)   Performed at 16–20 weeks gestation; results available in 4 weeks
    (ii) Procedural fetal mortality = 0.3%
    (iii) Late abortion required
3. Chorionic villus sampling with DNA analysis:
    (i)   Performed at 9–11 weeks gestation; results available in 3–4 weeks
    (ii) Procedural fetal mortality = 4%
    (iii) Allows first trimester abortion

DNA analysis

Small amounts of DNA can be amplified using the polymerase chain reaction (PCR):
1. Restriction endonuclease mapping—identifies molecular lesion, e.g. inversion/deletion
2. Restriction fragment length polymorphism (RFLP) linkage analysis—determines chromosome carrying abnormal gene
3. Oligonucleotide probes—detect specific mutation

B. ACQUIRED HAEMOLYTIC ANAEMIAS

HAEMOLYTIC (ISOIMMUNE) DISEASE OF THE NEWBORN

Pathogenesis

1. Passage of Rhesus (Rh) positive fetal red cells into the maternal (Rh-negative) circulation with consequent immunisation

2. Production of IgG isoantibodies (then or in later pregnancies)
3. Transplacental transfer of antibodies which may destroy fetal red cells in utero (of increasing significance with further pregnancies and Rhesus-positive fetuses)
4. ABO incompatability may similarly result in the production of antibodies (of less clinical significance)
5. Alternative means of immunisation—previous transfusion of Rh-positive blood into Rh-negative female
6. Degrees of haemolysis and compensation in the fetus and newborn
7. Unconjugated bilirubin >340 µmol/l may produce neurological damage postnatally, especially to the basal nuclei (kernicterus)

Haematology
1. Hb levels may be normal or very low (with cord blood levels <5 g/dl)
2. Reticulocytosis (up to 70%) and erythroblastosis (with many more nucleated cells than WBC in severe cases)
3. Neutrophilia, usual with active haemolysis
4. In ABO incompatibility—milder abnormalities, e.g. spherocytes in the blood film
5. Serology:
   (i) With Rh incompatability—positive direct Coombs test due to anti-D antibodies
   (ii) With ABO incompatability—direct Coombs test usually only weakly positive or negative

Clinical features
The physical findings depend on the severity of the haemolytic process:
1. Massive generalised oedema (hydrops fetalis) in severe cases
2. Variable anaemia
3. Jaundice—appears within the first 24 hours, maximum on day 3–4
4. Hepatosplenomegaly
5. Kernicterus:
   (i) Early—hypotonia, lethargy, poor feeding
   (ii) Later—hypertonia with head retraction, death. Surviving infants have neurological defects

Treatment
1. Prevention:
   (i) All Rh(D)-negative mothers of Rh (D)-positive infants should be given 500 iu anti-D immunoglobulin within 72 hours of delivery
   (ii) Mothers requiring additional doses to cover transplacental bleeds of >4 ml identified by Kleihauer test (for detection of

fetal RBC in maternal circulation)—125 iu anti-D per ml RBC required

   (iii) Abortion, amniocentesis, external cephalic version, chorionic villus sampling—250 iu anti-D (less than 20 weeks gestation) or 500 iu anti-D (more than 20 weeks)
   (iv) For accidental transfusion of Rh (D)-negative female of child-bearing age with Rh(D)-positive blood—25 000 iu anti-D/unit blood
   (v) In first pregnancy antenatal prophylaxis prevents primary immunisation

2. Where sensitisation has occurred and Rh haemolytic disease is anticipated (increased maternal anti-D titres; bile pigments in amniotic fluid serially measured spectrophotometrically predict disease severity and progression):
   (i) Maternal antenatal plasma exchange
   (ii) Intrauterine transfusion at 18–24 weeks
   (iii) Planned premature delivery after 30 weeks
   (iv) Exchange transfusion if cord Hb $\leq$ 12 g/dl and/or bilirubin $\geq$ 68 μmol/l
   (v) Phototherapy for milder cases with neonatal jaundice

ACQUIRED AUTOIMMUNE HAEMOLYTIC ANAEMIA

Classification

1. Primary or 'idiopathic'—over half of all patients at diagnosis
2. Secondary or 'associated'—the majority of cases when fully investigated or after a period of observation

Pathogenesis

1. Production of proteins, usually IgG immunoglobulins, which act as antibodies active at normal body temperature and damage the red cell membrane
2. Alternatively antibodies, usually IgM immunoglobulins, which act as cold agglutinins, interacting with complement and damaging red cells at lower temperatures
3. Damaged red cells lose their deformability and are subject to fragmentation, with the production of spherocytes
4. Premature destruction of red cells

Haematology

1. Variable anaemia; macrocytosis may reflect reticulocytosis and/or frequently associated folate deficiency
2. Reticulocytosis—correlates quite well with severity of the haemolysis when marrow function is not compromised
3. Blood film—spherocytes and poikilocytes (sometimes bizarre)
4. Bone marrow—erythroid hyperplasia; may show degrees of megaloblastic change

5. Serology:
   (i) 'Warm' antibody active at 37°C—direct Coombs (antiglobulin) test usually positive (where the reagent has broad-spectrum anti-IgG and anti-complement specificities)
   (ii) 'Cold' antibody, which fixes to red cells at low temperatures (e.g. 4°C)—positive direct Coombs test of anti-complement specificity, often with anti-I specificity

Biochemistry
The non-specific features of haemolysis (see p. 16).

Clinical features
1. May occur at any age, though 'cold' agglutinin associated disease is chiefly seen in middle and old age
2. The onset is usually insidious but may be dramatically acute with evidence of intravascular haemolysis
3. Symptoms are often minimal but acute haemolysis may produce:
   (i) Fever
   (ii) Pain in abdomen/back
   (iii) Rapidly developing jaundice
4. With 'cold' antibodies, symptoms are often aggravated by exposure to cold (Raynaud's phenomenon may also occur)
5. Variable jaundice (reflecting the degree of haemolysis and the functional capacity of the liver)
6. Splenomegaly–in over 50% of patients
7. Features of the associated disease may predominate

Associations
1. Haematological malignancies:
   (i) Leukaemias—notably chronic lymphocytic leukaemia
   (ii) Lymphomas
2. Collagen disease, e.g. SLE
3. Drug ingestion:
   (i) Methyldopa—probably due to stimulated antibody (IgG) formation, the reaction does *not* require the presence of the drug. In patients who receive methyldopa, a positive Coombs test is common, significant haemolysis infrequent
   (ii) Penicillin (in large doses)—acts as a hapten, binds to red cell membrane and stimulates the production of IgG antibody
   (iii) Quinine and quinidine—due to IgM antibody and immune complex formation ('innocent bystander' mechanism) which secondarily causes the activation of complement. Can cause acute intravascular lysis
4. Infections:
   (i) *Mycoplasma* pneumonia, also various viral infections, e.g.

infectious mononucleosis—due to IgM antibodies which act as cold agglutinins. Brisk haemolytic episodes usually occur 2–3 weeks after the clinical manifestations of infection

(ii) Syphilis, also various viral infections—due to the Donath–Landsteiner (IgG) antibody which fixes to red cells at low temperatures but only produces haemolysis at 37°C. Causes acute haemolysis with paroxysmal cold haemoglobinuria

Treatment
1. Of the associated disease state — not uniformly successful, i.e. the haemolytic process may require treatment as separate entity
2. Withdrawal of drug (though the Coombs test may remain positive for months/years in the methyldopa type)
3. Corticosteroids—principally for warm antibody types. The majority of patients respond
4. Immunosuppressive/cytotoxic drug therapy, e.g. azathioprine, cyclophosphamide or chlorambucil (particularly when steroids alone fail)
5. Splenectomy—in resistant cases or where high steroid dosage has had to be continued (for 'warm' antibody, idiopathic types, rather than secondary)
6. Supportive:
   (i) Transfusions should be avoided if possible (accurate cross-matching is impossible) but are sometimes life-saving
   (ii) In 'cold' agglutinin associated disease—warm clothing and avoidance of exposure to cold; transfuse via blood warmer

ACQUIRED NON-IMMUNE HAEMOLYTIC ANAEMIA

Red cells may be damaged and their life-span significantly reduced in a variety of ways and by a number of agents.

1. Chemical agents and physical factors
(i) Heavy metals, e.g. lead (also directly impairs erythropoiesis, see p. 42)
(ii) Arsine gas (by-product of metal refining)
(iii) Sodium and potassium chlorate—an oxidative effect
(iv) Snake venom and insect poisons
(v) Excessive temperature (e.g. in severe burns), excessive haemodilution, breathing 100% oxygen
(vi) Hypophosphataemia—decreases phosphates in red cells and impairs glycolysis; a complication of incorrect i.v. feeding

2. Mechanical damage ('fragmented red cell syndromes')
(i)   Cardiac valvular disease—notably by replacement valves (e.g. Starr–Edwards) but rarely in calcific disease. Most patients compensate adequately for the haemolysis
(ii) In disseminated intravascular coagulation (DIC) (see also p. 140):
 a. Pathology—red cells are 'sheared' on fibrin strands; the resulting 'schistocytes' are rigid and metabolically compromised
 b. Many clinical associations—notably severe infections, malignant disease and microangiopathies (e.g. in malignant hypertension, collagenoses and obstetric pathologies)
(iii) March haemoglobinuria—red cells are principally damaged in circulation through the soles of the feet—usually as a result of prolonged walking, route marching, running

3. Drug ingestion
Red cells are susceptible to damage by oxidative drugs and especially if G-6-PD-deficient; e.g. dapsone invariably causes haemolysis, the antimalarial primaquine only causes haemolysis in G-6-PD-deficient patients.

4. Infection
(i)   Invasion of red cells by microorganisms, e.g. malaria, oroya fever (due to *Bartonella bacilliformis*)
(ii) Damage to red cell membrane by toxins, e.g. *Clostridium welchii*

5. Paroxysmal nocturnal haemoglobinuria (PNH)
(i)   A rare condition of 3rd–5th decades
(ii) Probably not a single entity, it may occur in association with haematological malignancies and dysplasias; clonal disorder
(iii) The defect—deficiency of decay accelerating factor (DAF) which inactivates red-cell-bound C_3a—results in sensitivity of red cell membrane to lysis by complement, especially in the lower pH range (basis of diagnostic Ham's test)
(iv) Bone marrow—may be hypoplastic (*conversely* PNH may develop in aplastic anaemia, see p. 53)
(v)   No specific therapy. Iron supplements may be required. Transfusions should be of washed or filtered red cells. Thrombotic problems require long-term anticoagulant treatment

FURTHER ADVANCED READING

Bunn H F, Forget B G 1985 Haemoglobin: molecular, genetic and clinical aspects. W B Saunders, Philadelphia

Dacie J V 1985 The haemolytic anaemias, 3rd edn. Churchill Livingstone, Edinburgh, vol. 1
Dacie J V 1988 The haemolytic anaemias, 3rd edn. Churchill Livingstone, Edinburgh, vol. 2
Serjeant G R 1985 Sickle cell disease. Oxford University Press, Oxford
Weatherall D J, Clegg J B 1992 The thalassaemia syndromes, 4th edn. Blackwell, Oxford

5. The porphyrias, lead poisoning and methaemoglobinaemia

Although rarely encountered, some knowledge of the basic features of these conditions is required.

THE PORPHYRIAS AND DISORDERS OF HAEM

THE PORPHYRIAS

Definition
Rare disorders of porphyrin metabolism in which there is tissue accumulation or increased excretion (or both) of porphyrins or porphyrin precursors.

'Erythropoietic' forms

1. Congenital erythropoietic porphyria
(i) Autosomal recessive transmission
(ii) Excessive production and accumulation of type I porphyrins (due to deficiency of uroporphyrinogen III co-synthetase)
(iii) Excess excretion of uroporphyrin I and coproporphyrin I in urine and faeces
(iv) Haemolysis (light destroys porphyrin-rich cells)
(v) Clinical features—disfiguring bullous dermatitis, induced by sunlight, fluorescent teeth and red urine, hirsutism and splenomegaly
(vi) Treatment—avoidance of sunlight, splenectomy and hypertransfusion with chelation (to completely suppress erythropoiesis)

2. Erythropoietic protoporphyria
(i) Autosomal dominant transmission
(ii) Protoporphyrin III is increased in red cells, plasma, liver and faeces (due to ferrochelatase deficiency)
(iii) Normal haematology
(iv) Clinical features—skin lesions induced by light, cirrhosis and hepatic failure
(v) Treatment—avoidance of sunlight; β carotene may reduce photosensitivity

'Hepatic' forms

1. Acute intermittent porphyria
(i)   Autosomal dominant transmission
(ii) Excess of porphobilinogen and uroporphyrin III in urine (may
      be dark red, especially after exposure to sunlight)
(iii) Normal haematology
(iv) Clinical features include intermittent abdominal pain

2. Cutaneous hepatic porphyria (various forms)
Normal haematology.

LEAD POISONING

Now uncommon. The incidence of 'domestic' cases (e.g. due to
lead contaminated water and lead paint) has considerably
decreased. 'Industrial' cases are still reported (e.g. in workers
involved in plastics manufacture and the destruction of old car
batteries).

Pathogenesis (of haematological changes)
1. Interference with normal haem synthesis, principally by
   inhibition of ALA synthetase, ALA dehydrase and haem
   synthetase (see p.166)
2. Abnormal erythropoiesis—production of defective red cells with
   basophilic stippling, abnormal membrane and a reduced life-
   span due to inhibition of pyrimidine 5-nucleotidase

Haematology
1. Anaemia—usually hypochromic, normocytic
2. Slight reticulocytosis
3. Blood film—basophilic stippling of red cells. Occasionally,
   nucleated red cells
4. Bone marrow—erythroid hyperplasia. Sideroblastic change may
   be seen

Biochemistry
1. Increased quantities of δ-aminolaevulinic acid and
   coproporphyrins in urine
2. Increased free protoporphyrin and coproporphyrin in red cells
3. Increased blood and urinary lead

Clinical features
Classically:
1. Lead line on gums (Burton's line)
2. Abdominal colic, constipation
3. Neuromuscular abnormalities, e.g. foot/wrist drop
4. Encephalopathy

METHAEMOGLOBINAEMIA

Basic features of methaemoglobin

1. Formation by oxidation of iron in haem from ferrous to ferric state
2. Inability to bind oxygen reversibly and therefore of no value in oxygen transport
3. Formation is prevented by:
   (i) Reducing agents—reduced glutathione and ascorbic acid
   (ii) An enzymatic mechanism—electron transport (by diaphorase) from NADH, produced by glycolysis
   (iii) Another enzymatic mechanism, requiring the presence of a redox dye, e.g. methylene blue—electron transport from NADPH, produced by pentose phosphate shunt (see p.19)
4. Formation is enhanced in infants—fetal haemoglobin is more susceptible to oxidation, reducing mechanisms are less efficient
5. Diagnostic spectral properties—the basis of optical density method of assay
6. Normally comprises < 1% of total haemoglobin
7. When > 10% of total haemoglobin, causes cyanosis; when >35% may cause hypoxic symptoms

CONGENITAL METHAEMOGLOBINAEMIA

Causes

1. *Enzymatic deficiencies (e.g. of diaphorase)*
   (i) Methaemoglobin 15–40%
   (ii) Potentially hazardous in infancy because of hypoxia; subsequently, asymptomatic cyanosis
   (iii) Reducing agents, e.g. methylene blue, ascorbic acid, ameliorate

2. *Haemoglobinopathies*
   (i) Unstable haemoglobins—rarely cause cyanosis (see p.27)
   (ii) Haemoglobin M disease—due to abnormal molecular configuration (*not* true methaemoglobinaemia, see p.27)

ACQUIRED METHAEMOGLOBINAEMIA

Causes

Drugs or their metabolites which act as oxidising agents.
Examples:
1. Nitrites, usually formed as a result of bacterial reduction of nitrates, e.g. in spinach
2. Aromatic nitro- or amino-compounds such as aniline dyes (when used to mark clothing, nappies) and phenacetin

Clinical features
1. Clinically significant changes, chiefly in new-born and infants
2. Cyanosis
3. Dyspnoea, lethargy, headaches
4. Acute intravascular haemolysis ± renal failure, e.g. arsine or sodium chlorate overdose

Treatment
1. Withdrawal of the offending agents (methaemoglobinaemia resolves in 1–2 days)
2. In the severely affected, injection of methylene blue

6. Secondary anaemias

Basic features
1. Anaemia is a frequent association of many primarily non-haematological disease states
2. The principal underlying causes are:
   (i) Depressed erythropoiesis (mechanisms differ)
   (ii) Poor iron utilisation in erythropoiesis
3. The anaemia is normochromic/hypochromic and normocytic/microcytic (macrocytosis is *usually* due to associated B_{12}/folate deficiency)
4. Patients affected are often treated with haematinics, e.g. iron, folate and vitamin B_{12}, to little or no effect—the anaemias may be labelled 'refractory' or due to 'malabsorption'

The most important examples and particular features are described.

IN RENAL INSUFFICIENCY

Pathogenesis
Not fully elucidated—erythropoiesis is depressed (probably due to impaired erythropoietic stimulation).
   Additional complicating factors:
1. Iron deficiency, especially in maintenance dialysis patients (blood loss plus dietary lack)
2. Folate deficiency (dietary lack plus loss in dialysate)
3. Aluminium toxicity (dialysis patients)

Haematology
1. Anaemia (uncomplicated by dominant iron/folate deficiencies) usually correlates well with blood urea/creatinine
2. Indices—MCHC, MCH and MCV usually normal; MCV *may* be reduced (e.g. iron-deficient dialysis patient)
3. Leucopenia—following dialysis, due to leucocyte adhesion to dialysis membrane
4. Blood film—red cells initially normal; with more severe anaemia, 'burr' cells and schistocytes

5. Platelet function commonly abnormal, with prolonged bleeding time—corrected by dialysis, cryoprecipitate or DDAVP
6. Bone marrow—often not grossly abnormal, sometimes hypoplastic; iron stores may be increased, normal or depleted

Biochemistry
1. Serum iron and TIBC frequently *both* decreased (poor correlation with iron status)
2. Reduced serum erythropoietin level (impaired renal production)

Treatment
1. Of renal disease—when possible, improvement in renal function ± dialysis
2. Blood transfusions—of transient value (most patients adapt to anaemia with shift in oxyhaemoglobin dissociation curve, see p.172)
3. Recombinant human erythropoietin (principal application in anaemia of chronic renal failure)
4. Correction of any associated nutritional deficiency

IN LIVER DISEASE

Pathogenesis
1. Liver disease in itself causes depression of erythropoiesis
2. 'Hypersplenism'—principally by increase in plasma volume
Additional complicating factors:
1. Iron deficiency due to blood loss (e.g. from varices)
2. Folate deficiency, chiefly dietary

Haematology (uncomplicated)
1. Indices—MCHC, MCH and MCV usually normal (may be slight macrocytosis)
2. Thrombocytopenia due to hypersplenism, folate deficiency, alcoholism or, rarely, DIC
3. Blood film:
   (i) Red cells which *appear* macrocytic ('leptocytes'), with increased diameter/thickness ratio due to increased membrane lipid and which usually also have appearance of target cells
   (ii) Acanthocytes/'spur' cells—less common but also related to membrane changes
4. Bone marrow—variable quantitative changes
5. Abnormal coagulation due to impaired synthesis of factors, vitamin K deficiency, dysfibrinogenaemia

Treatment
1. Of liver disease
2. Splenectomy—sometimes indicated and beneficial
3. Of any associated nutritional deficiency

IN ALCOHOLISM

Pathogenesis
Alcohol has a *direct* effect on haematopoiesis, especially
erythropoiesis, which is impaired.
   Additional factors:
1. Nutritional deficiencies, notably of folate
2. Liver disease, with or without hypersplenism due to portal
   hypertension
3. Blood loss (varices)
4. Intravascular haemolysis associated with fatty change in the
   liver, and elevated plasma triglyceride/cholesterol
   levels—Zieve's syndrome

Haematology
(1) Indices—MCV often slightly increased (marked increase
    usually indicates associated folate deficiency)
(2) Blood film—typically round macrocyte (cf. oval in B_{12} / folate
    deficiency)
(3) Bone marrow—characteristic vacuolisation of erythroid
    precursors. Sideroblastic change, which is reversible, may be
    seen

Treatment
Withdrawal of alcohol.

IN CHRONIC INFECTION AND/OR INFLAMMATION

Pathogenesis
1. Depressed erythropoiesis
2. Poor iron utilisation
Additional complicating factors:
1. Nutritional deficiencies, especially of folate (requirements
   increase, intake often falls)
2. Blood loss, e.g. due to anti-inflammatory drugs in rheumatoid
   arthritis

Haematology (uncomplicated)
1. Indices—MCHC, MCH and MCV may be normal or decreased
   (depending on the relative importance of poor iron utilisation in
   the production of anaemia)
2. Blood film—mild hypochromia is common
3. Bone marrow—non-specific quantitative changes. Iron stores
   are often normal or increased but normal sideroblasts are

reduced (abnormal sideroblasts may be seen and 'rings' in secondary sideroblastic change)
4. Ferrokinetic studies (^{59}Fe) confirm decreased iron utilisation in haemoglobin synthesis

Biochemistry
Serum iron and TIBC *both* decreased (see Fig. 2.1, p.6).
  Ferritin—may be normal or increased (acute phase reactant).

Associations
1. Chronic infections—e.g. bronchiectasis, osteomyelitis, bacterial endocarditis
2. Inflammatory disease—e.g. Crohn's disease, rheumatoid arthritis

Treatment
Of the associated disease.

IN MALIGNANCY

Pathogeneis
1. Depressed erythropoiesis
2. Poor iron utilisation
Additional complicating factors:
1. Nutritional deficiencies
2. Blood loss
3. Marrow invasion by metastases (producing leuco-erythroblastic anaemia)
4. DIC

Haematology
Similar to that seen in chronic infection/inflammation.

Treatment
While there may be correctable factors, some degree of anaemia usually persists.

IN HYPOTHYROIDISM

Pathogeneis
Decreased metabolic rate results in reduced erythropoietic requirement.
  Additional complicating factors:
1. B$_{12}$ deficiency (due to Addisonian pernicious anaemia)
2. Iron ± folate deficiency (due to dietary lack—'loss of interest', or blood loss due to menorrhagia)

Haematology (uncomplicated)
1. Anaemia—mild/moderate, normochromic, normocytic
2. Bone marrow—relatively hypoplastic

Treatment
1. Thyroid replacement therapy
2. Haematinics, e.g. B_{12}, if indicated

IN HYPOPITUITARISM

Reduced red cell mass related to hormonal deficiencies—returns to normal with hormonal replacement therapy.

IN PREGNANCY

1. Dilutional anaemia —disproportionate increase in plasma volume (50%) cf. RBC mass (20–30%)
2. Iron ± folate deficiency—requires correction

7. Aplastic anaemia

APLASTIC/HYPOPLASTIC ANAEMIA

Definition
Reduction in haemopoietic tissue, not a consequence of bone marrow fibrosis or malignant infiltration, resulting in peripheral blood cytopenias.

Classification
1. Severe (SAA)—10% chance of recovery:
   (i) Pancytopenia with at least two of the following:
       a. Neutrophils $< 0.5 \times 10^9/l$ (VSAA if $< 0.2 \times 10^9/l$)
       b. Platelets $< 20 \times 10^9/l$
       c. Reticulocytes $< 1\%$
   (ii) Trephine biopsy:
       a. Severely hypocellular ($< 25\%$ normal) or
       b. Moderately hypocellular (25–50% normal) with $< 30\%$ of remaining cells haemopoietic
2. Non-severe (NSAA)— 50% chance of recovery

Basic features
There are two fundamentally different types.

1. Predictable, often rapidly reversible, hypoplasia
(i) Usually a consequence of ionising radiation and/or cytotoxic chemotherapy. Dose-dependent
(ii) Rapidly dividing maturing haemopoietic cells are principally affected rather than pluripotent stem cells
But
(iii) Repeated or prolonged therapy may deplete the stem cell compartment and cause chronic hypoplasia

2. Unpredictable, often irreversible hypoplasia
(i) Primary 'idiopathic' or secondary to 'idiosyncratic' reactions to drugs or virus infections
(ii) Probably chiefly due to haemopoietic stem cell defect/ damage

(iii) May sometimes be related to auto-immune phenomena or changes in the micro-environment of stem cells

(iv) Chronic reduction in number *or* functional capacity of stem cells

Some types of aplasia, including childhood forms, have particular characteristics as discussed on p.53.

Pathogenesis

1. Reduction in haemopoietic tissue and increase in fat spaces in bone marrow
2. Deficient cell production, usually reflected firstly in granulocyte and platelet counts
3. Typically, development of pancytopenia

Haematology

1. Anaemia—normocytic or macrocytic, normochromic
2. Reticulocytopenia usual (*absolute* counts more reliable)
3. Leucopenia:
   (i) Granulocytes often $< 1.5 \times 10^9/l$ (mature, but may show 'toxic' granulation with high LAP score)
   (ii) Lymphopenia may occur, with relative and absolute decrease in T cells, significance uncertain
4. Thrombocytopenia—platelets often $< 30 \times 10^9/l$, morphologically normal
5. HbF may be increased, especially in childhood disease
6. Bone marrow:
   (i) Hypocellular—residual haemopoietic tissue often unevenly distributed (an aspirate may provide a misleading, cellular specimen—histology of a biopsy gives a better overall picture of degree of hypocellularity)
   (ii) Iron stores increased, especially in repeatedly transfused patients
   (iii) Increased macrophage activity ± haemophagocytosis

Biochemistry

1. Plasma iron often increased, TIBC normal or decreased and percentage saturation increased
2. Plasma ^{55}Fe clearance prolonged, utilisation for haemoglobin synthesis reduced

Clinical features

1. Uncommon, but increasing in frequency—3–$6/10^6$ population per annum in developed countries
2. About 70% of all cases are 'idiopathic' without known associations (see below)
3. May occur at any age

4. Mode of onset varies from insidious to dramatic
5. Presentation—commonly with haemorrhage (e.g. purpura, petechiae) due to thrombocytopenia
6. Symptoms and signs reflecting neutropenia – oral ulceration, infections
7. Symptoms and signs due to anaemia
8. Hepato-splenomegaly/lymphadenopathy *not* characteristic

Associations
1. Drug ingestion (other than anti-cancer chemotherapy):
    (i)   Antibiotic—chloramphenicol, sulphonamides
    (ii) Anti-inflammatory—phenylbutazone, gold, indomethacin, benoxaprofen
    (iii) Anti-epileptic—hydantoin, trimethadione
    (iv) Anti-diabetic—chlorpropamide, tolbutamide
    (v)   Anti-thyroid—propylthiouracil, potassium perchlorate
    (iv) Psychotropic—chlorpromazine (transient)
2. Exposure to chemicals:
    (i)   Aromatic hydrocarbons—benzene
    (ii) Insecticides—gammabenzene hexachloride (Lindane)
    (iii) Aniline dyes
3. Infection:
    (i)   Viral—notably viral hepatitis (A, B and C), EBV, influenza A, HIV (? autoimmune reaction)
    (ii) Bacterial—miliary tuberculosis

Treatment
Depends on disease severity, patient's age and availability of HLA-matched BMT donor.
1. Removal of associated factors—e.g. withdrawal of causal drugs
2. Supportive:
    (i)   Red cell transfusions ⎫ Should be filtered to minimise
    (ii) Platelet transfusions ⎬ HLA sensitisation, and CMV-negative if patient is CMV-negative
    (iii) Antibiotics
    (iv) Prophylactic antifungal mouth-care ± gut sterilisation
    (v)   Protective isolation—single room with reversed barrier nursing
3. Bone marrow transplantation (BMT)—treatment of choice for young patients with SAA and HLA identical donor.
    Rejection rates are increased in patients given transfusions pre-BMT
4. Immunosuppression:
    (i)   Antilymphocyte/antithymocyte globulin (ALG/ATG) — of horse or rabbit origin — may counter immunological suppression.

Side-effects — anaphylaxis; serum sickness with fever, rash and arthralgia 1– 3 weeks after treatment; antiplatelet activity with worsening of haemorrhagic tendency

50 – 60% response rate

(ii) High-dose methylprednisolone—20 mg/kg/d × 3, followed by reducing regime. May be beneficial if no response to ALG

(iii) Cyclosporin A—promising responses reported; subject of therapeutic studies

5. Androgens (e.g. 17 alkylated androgens, oxymethalone):
    (i) May take 2–3 months to achieve response
    (ii) Recovery is usually independent of continuing 'maintenance' therapy
    (iii) May be used with ALG
    (iv) Side-effects - virilisation, prostatic enlargement, salt retention, hepatocellular carcinoma, and peliosis hepatis

6. Growth factors:
    GM-CSF
    G-CSF   } may be of value—under
    Interleukin 3   investigation

Prognosis

Varies considerably.

Bone marrow transplantation gives 50% long-term survival, with greatest mortality in first year. Immunosuppression gives 50% long-term survival, with risk of late complications, including development of paroxysmal nocturnal haemoglobinuria (PNH), myelodysplasia or acute leukaemia.

SPECIAL TYPES OF APLASIA

1. Fanconi's anaemia

(i) Hereditary—rare autosomal recessive

(ii) Anaemia, macrocytic. Insidious in onset—usually presents at about the age of 5

(iii) Associated with cytogenetic and multiple physical anomalies, e.g. skin pigmentation, skeletal defects, microcephaly, growth retardation, renal abnormalities

(iv) Poor prognosis—10% develop AML

(v) Treatment—supportive, BMT, androgens

2. Associated with paroxysmal nocturnal haemoglobinuria (PNH)

(i) PNH usually develops a variable time after the hypoplasia —possibly due to emergence of mutant stem cell clone

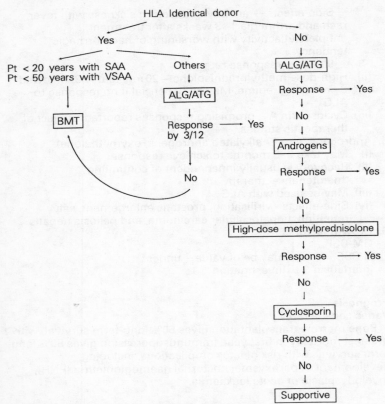

Fig. 7.1 Treatment of severe aplastic anaemia

(ii) Alternatively, an episode of hypoplasia may occur in a patient who has PNH with haemolysis (see p.39)
(iii) Acidified serum lysis test (Ham's test)—positive
(iv) No specific therapy. Supportive treatment

3. Red cell aplasia (selective depression of the erythroid series)
(i) Blackfan–Diamond syndrome (congenital)—anaemia, macrocytic. Presents typically within first year. Often responds to corticosteroids, though spontaneous remissions occur
(ii) Acquired:
   a. Acute—'aplastic crisis' in haemolytic anaemia (associations include B_{19} parvovirus infection and post-rubella). May respond to folic acid

b. Chronic—the majority are associated with thymomas or a
   recognisable auto-immune disease (e.g. SLE)
   Thymectomy and/or immunosuppressant drugs are often
   beneficial

FURTHER ADVANCED READING

Gordon Smith E C (ed) 1989. Clinical haematology. Baillière Tindall, London,
   vol 2:1

8. Hypersplenism

Basic concepts
1. Splenomegaly occurs in many conditions but hypersplenism is not necessarily associated with all of these
2. The principal normal functions of the spleen are:
   (i) Haematopoiesis in fetal life—limited to formation of lymphoid cells and monocytes after birth
   (ii) Removal of old or defective blood cells (especially red cells) from the circulation
   (iii) Removal ('pitting') of red cell inclusions (e.g. Howell–Jolly bodies, siderotic granules) and modification of the red cell membrane (e.g. reduction in lipid content)
   (iv) Cell reservoir—chiefly of platelets, (30–40% of platelet mass). The splenic red cell mass is relatively small in man
   (v) Production of immunoglobulins—antibodies
   (vi) Modulation of haematopoiesis in the marrow by ill-defined mechanisms
   (vii) Phagocytosis of (encapsulated) bacteria
3. Hypersplenism is best defined as reduction in red cell, granulocyte or platelet count, despite normal marrow production, as a result of:
   (i) Exaggerated sequestration of old or defective cells
   (ii) Sequestration of normal cells—stasis of increased numbers of cells in an enlarged spleen results in metabolic stress and premature removal from circulation
   (iii) Expansion of plasma volume (in itself a cause of *relative* cytopenias)
Note: Sometimes a variety of immunological disease states, haemolytic anaemias and ITP are cited as examples of 'hypersplenism'—a more restricted and therefore less unwieldy use of the term is applied here

Causes/associations
1. Portal hypertension (congestive splenomegaly usually with cirrhosis of the liver)
2. Rheumatoid arthritis (Felty's syndrome)
3. Malignant lymphomas (immunological mechanisms/bone

marrow invasion may be of more relevance in producing blood changes)
4. Infections/infestations—tuberculosis, syphilis, leishmaniasis (kala azar), malaria (sometimes labelled 'tropical splenomegaly')
5. Sarcoidosis
6. Gaucher's disease
7. Lipid storage disease (e.g. Niemann–Pick disease)
8. Idiopathic
9. Miscellaneous—variably significant hypersplenism is seen in a number of haematological disease states, especially where blood transfusions are given in supportive therapy, e.g. myeloproliferative disorders, thalassaemia. The hypersplenism often increases transfusion requirements, but dissociation from the effects of the disease per se can be difficult

Clinical features
1. Those relating to associated disease
2. Splenomegaly—the spleen is usually, but not invariably, readily palpable

Treatment
1. Of underlying cause or associated disease—often has little or no effect on hypersplenism
2. Splenectomy—the likely benefits and possible hazards must be weighed carefully. Decisions depend on:
   (i)   The severity of the cytopenias
   (ii) The associated disease state
   (iii) The general state of the patient
3. Consequences of splenectomy:
   (i)   Reduction in plasma volume to normal or near normal
   (ii) Red cells—appearance in film of target cells, cells with nuclear remnants (e.g. Howell–Jolly bodies) and siderocytes (i.e. cells no longer removed/modified by the spleen)
   (iii) White cells—early increase in neutrophils, within hours, and subsequent fall towards normal with increase in lymphocytes
   (iv) Platelets—early increase, within hours, and subsequent fall towards normal (within a few months)
   (v)   Increased susceptibility to infection, especially pneumococcus, meningococcus, *H. influenzae* and *E. coli*, notably in children. Pneumococcal vaccine given pre-splenectomy and prophylactic antibiotics (e.g. penicillin V 250 mg b.d.) post-splenectomy are appropriate counter measures
4. Failed splenectomy—the persistence or recurrence of hypersplenism suggests an incorrect diagnosis or the presence of an accessory spleen

HYPOSPLENISM

Blood changes similar to the post-splenectomy picture are seen in:
1. Congenital absence of the spleen
2. Splenic atrophy, e.g. in coeliac disease, dermatitis herpetiformis, ulcerative colitis, Crohn's disease, and in sickle cell disease ('autosplenectomy' due to repeated infarction)

9. Lymphoproliferative disorders

MALIGNANT LYMPHOPROLIFERATIVE DISEASES

Basic concepts

1. Lymphoid cells mature and develop competence in the bursa/bone marrow (B cells) or thymus (T cells)
2. Subsequent sequences of differentiation/transformation in lymph nodes are influenced by antigenic stimuli (antigen-dependent phase)
3. A useful working concept of the lymphoproliferative diseases is that the predominant cell is the equivalent of an 'arrested' stage in the maturation and differentiation of lymphocytes
4. Proliferations in which malignant precursor cells predominate are the B and T lymphoblastic lymphomas
5. Proliferations corresponding to more mature cell types are diverse. B-cell diseases span chronic lymphatic leukaemia, most non-Hodgkin's lymphomas and myelomatosis. T-cell diseases represent a wide spectrum (increasingly so with identification of clonality)
6. While some diseases represent fairly well defined entities pathologically and clinically, others, notably the non-Hodgkin's lymphomas, are heterogenous
7. The malignant proliferations are clonal, arising from a single cell type
8. Monoclonality is indicated by the presence of:
   (i) one light chain type, κ or λ (kappa or lambda) in surface-associated or secreted immunoglobulin/paraprotein
   (ii) unique antigenic specificity due to rearrangements of the genes coding for cell surface immunoglobulin/T-cell receptor
9. Immunological marker studies are resulting in the recognition of many subsets within the broader categories
10. The majority of lymphoproliferative disorders appear to have multifactorial aetiology with genetic and immunological components; there are some with specific viral aetiological links

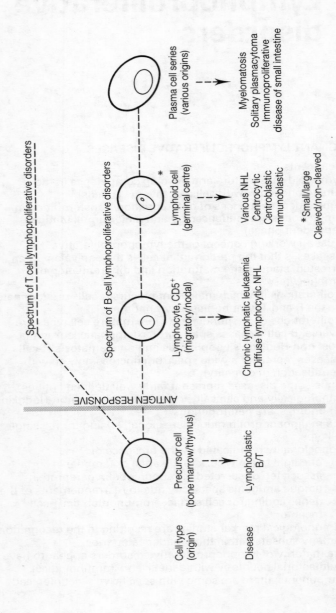

Fig. 9.1 Cell origin of lymphoproliferative diseases

11. Cells of non-lymphoid origin, e.g. histiocytes, may (rarely) be the origin of the malignant clone and may be included as 'lymphomas'

CHRONIC LYMPHOCYTIC LEUKAEMIA (CLL)

Pathology
1. Progressive accumulation of lymphocytic cells in sites where lymphocytes normally occur (initially without appreciable disturbance of normal architecture)
2. In the great majority of cases these are B lymphocytes (T-cell CLL is very rare)
3. The infiltration of bone marrow results in compromised marrow function as the disease progresses
4. The lymphocytes in CLL are immunologically incompetent

Haematology
1. Anaemia—normocytic, normochromic—often develops as the disease progresses. A Coombs-positive haemolytic anaemia may occur (10–20%)
2. Lymphocytosis—$>5 \times 10^9/l$, often $>50 \times 10^9/l$, occasionally $>250 \times 10^9/l$
3. Thrombocytopenia is a feature of advanced disease
4. Blood film—lymphocytes are usually seen as:
   (i)   Small cells with densely clumped nuclear chromatin and a narrow rim of cytoplasm (predominant)
   (ii) Larger cells with lighter cytoplasm
   (iii) Smear or 'basket' cells—bare lymphocyte nuclei
5. Bone marrow—increased percentage of lymphocytes (>25%; often >75%)

Immunology
1. Surface immunoglobulin (SIg) is usually IgM or IgM + IgD
2. Serum immunoglobulin levels (notably IgM) are reduced in over 50% of patients, reflecting the functional defects of CLL lymphocytes
3. Antibody responses to infections are impaired
4. Paraproteinaemia (monoclonal gammopathy) ± Bence Jones (light chain) proteinuria—uncommon
5. CD5 antigen on cell surface in absence of other pan-T markers; Leu-1 positive, cALLA negative

Radiology
1. Lymphadenopathy may be detected at various sites (e.g. by CT scan)
2. Lytic bone lesions and/or more diffuse osteoporosis may be seen in advanced disease

Clinical features
1. A disease of middle and old age, predominantly in males
2. Often found 'incidentally' when blood tests are done for various reasons
3. The onset is insidious and progression slow
4. Some patients have *no* physical signs
5. Lymphadenopathy—often generalised and symmetrical with usually discrete, rubbery and painless (1–5 cm) nodes
6. Splenomegaly and hepatomegaly—frequently develop
7. Anaemia—initially mild but may be severe, with increasing weakness and dyspnoea. Important to consider autoimmune haemolysis (see p.36)
8. Haemorrhagic manifestations—in advanced disease
9. Recurrent infections, e.g. chest (reflecting immuno-suppression)
10. Skin lesions—due to lymphocytic infiltration or 'non-specific'
11. Systemic symptoms, e.g. sweats and weight loss—usually in advanced disease

Staging systems
Of value as an assessment of extent of disease ('tumour load') at the time of diagnosis and subsequently (especially in relation to treatment). One system which is in general use is that according to Binet:

Stage	Clinical features	Haematology
A	<3 sites involved (cervical/axillary/inguinal nodes, spleen, liver)	Hb $\geq$10 g/dl platelets $\geq$100 $\times$ 10^9/l
B	$\geq$3 sites involved (nodal $\pm$ spleen $\pm$ liver)	Hb $\geq$10 g/dl platelets $\geq$100 $\times$ 10^9/l
C	Not relevant to this stage	Hb <10 g/dl platelets <100 $\times$ 10^9/l

Treatment
1. No treatment is indicated for patients with stable, asymptomatic stage A disease
2. For more advanced disease and/or disease which shows progression:
   (i) Chemotherapy
      a. Single alkylating agent, usually chorambucil given intermittently, effective in reducing malignant cell load and stabilising disease in about 70% of cases
      b. Corticosteroids—chiefly as initial treatment where bone marrow function is compromised or for autoimmune complications

     c. Combination chemotherapy which includes an anthracycline is increasingly given as more 'vigorous' treatment to achieve greater cytoreduction and better short-term response; long-term benefit in terms of survival as yet uncertain
  (ii) Radiotherapy has a lesser role but can contribute to overall management
     a. To spleen, e.g. as intermittent low dose, reducing total tumour load and spleen size
     b. To nodes, e.g. if bulky, causing pressure symptoms and chemoresistant
3. Splenectomy—may be of value in patients not responding to other therapy and with splenomegaly as the only physical sign.
4. Supportive—infections, a reflection of the immunoparesis, require prompt and appropriate treatment with antibiotics; when immunoglobulin levels are particularly low, regular infusions of immunoglobulins, e.g. monthly, may be helpful as prophylaxis
5. More than one mode of therapy is often required during the course of the disease. Marrow depression is common and frequently limits the use of cytotoxic agents

Prognosis
1. Wide variation in the rate of progression of disease
2. Stage, age and response to treatment are prognostic indicators; women fare better than men
3. Overall prognosis is better than in any other leukaemia, over half of all patients surviving longer than 5 years and some over 15 years
4. Majority of deaths are disease-related, pulmonary infection being the commonest terminal event; non-CLL deaths are frequent in older patients

PROLYMPHOCYTIC LEUKAEMIA (PLL)

A rare disease which should, however, be distinguished from CLL.

Pathology
The characteristic cell has a large vesicular nucleolus and stains intensely for surface immuoglobulin.

Haematology
1. WBC increased, often markedly (> 100 × 10^9/l)
2. Blood film—prolymphocytes predominate
3. Bone marrow—prolymphocytic infiltration

Clinical features
1. Splenomegaly—early; usually becomes massive
   (*Note*: lymph node enlargement absent or inconspicuous)
2. Systemic symptoms

Course and prognosis
Responds less well (to chemotherapy) than CLL and survival is shorter.

HAIRY-CELL LEUKAEMIA (HCL OR LEUKAEMIC RETICULOENDOTHELIOSIS)

An atypical B-lymphoid malignancy (rare compared to CLL).

Pathology
1. Pathognomonic cell has predominantly lymphocytic characteristics (though is also 'monocytoid' and phagocytic)
2. Infiltration primarily involves bone marrow, spleen and liver
3. Bone marrow function is compromised
4. Degrees of hypersplenism develop

Haematology
1. Cytopenias/pancytopenia—common: monocytes often absent
2. Blood film—hairy cells, rarely very numerous (usually show positive tartrate-resistant acid phosphatase reaction)
3. Bone marrow—'dry-tap' common. Aspirate/imprint from trephine biopsy shows characteristic cell infiltration

Electron microscopy
Useful in visualisation of characteristic cytoplasmic villi and other features.

Biochemistry
Serum lysozyme level usually normal or low (contrasting with monocytic leukaemias).

Clinical features
1. A disease of middle and old age with male preponderance
2. Splenomegaly—usual; hepatomegaly occurs but lymphadenopathy is unusual
3. Sequelae of neutropenia—opportunistic infections

Treatment
1. Splenectomy — a standard first-line approach; usually results in marked improvement in blood counts and prolonged partial remission

2. Alpha interferon (α-interferon)—response rates of 70–90% (complete in 10–15%); maintenance therapy required and remissions not enduring. Toxicity varies but can preclude use
3. Deoxycoformycin—also achieves response rates of about 80% (complete remissions in the majority). Toxicity moderate; can induce marked immunosuppression; costly with limited availability
4. 2-chlorodeoxyadenosine (a deoxyadenosine analogue)— complete remission rate of 90% reported with short-term treatment (7-day infusion). May prove superior to any other form of treatment

Course and prognosis
1. Reflects the degree of severity of cytopenias, especially neutropenia (infective deaths common)
2. Median survival with current therapy—>5 years

SPLENIC LYMPHOMA WITH VILLOUS LYMPHOCYTES

A disease closely related to hairy-cell leukaemia but with a different response to treatment—unresponsive to α-interferon.

HODGKIN'S DISEASE (HD)

Aetiology
Unknown; possibility of an association with viral infection requires substantiation.

Pathology
1. Mixed cellular proliferation in which there are many non-neoplastic 'reactive' cells (lymphocytes, histiocytes, eosinophils)
2. Pathognomic malignant cells—the Reed–Sternberg cell, with distinctive bilobed nucleus with large prominent nucleoli—probably neoplastic form of activated lymphoid cell, T- or B-cell type
3. Histological classifications:
   (i) Lymphocyte predominant (LP), diffuse/nodular— comparable to low grade NHL; carries good prognosis
   (ii) Nodular sclerosis (NS), two categories—
      a. Type I—good prognosis
      b. Type II—poor prognosis
   (iii) Mixed cellularity (MC)—good prognosis
   (iv) Lymphocyte depleted (LD)—poor prognosis
4. These prognostic groupings are helpful but need to be considered together with other prognostic factors which may be more important (see below)

5. There may be progression from less to more aggressive histology, i.e. to LD
6. Principal mode of spread is directly via lymphatics (contrasts with NHL)
7. Occurrence of disease at multiple sites may be due to either dissemination or simultaneous proliferation
8. Defective cell-mediated immunity (e.g. impaired delayed hypersensitivity reaction)

Haematology
1. Often normal
2. Anaemia:
   (i)   Slight to moderate normochromic, normocytic (relating to the activity and extent of disease)
   (ii) Haemolytic anaemia infrequent (see p.36)
3. WBC:
   (i)   Neutrophilia—common
   (ii) Eosinophilia—occasionally a striking feature
   (iii) Lymphopenia—very common
4. Platelets—often increased in active disease
5. Blood film:
   (i)   Leuco-erythroblastic picture—occasional (a consequence of marrow infiltration)
   (ii) Circulating Reed–Sternberg cells—rare
6. ESR/plasma viscosity—a crude non-specific guide to disease activity
7. Bone marrow—usually non-specific. Trephine reveals HD in a minority of patients

Biochemistry
1. Non-specific protein changes—acute-phase reactant proteins, serum caeruloplasmin may reflect disease activity
2. Tests of liver, bone and renal function may be abnormal as a result of extensive disease or secondary effects

Imaging
1. Chest X-ray, e.g. demonstrating mediastinal nodal disease
2. Skeletal X-rays—osteolytic and osteoblastic lesions may occur principally in axial skeleton
3. Bipedal lymphography—demonstrates intra-abdominal nodal pattern well but increasingly replaced by scanning
4. Computed tomography (CT scan)—able to give whole-body assessment of disease extent
5. Ultrasonography—useful and relatively simple, best used as adjunctive procedure (valuable in identifying liver lesions)
6. Magnetic resonance imaging (MRI)—capable of providing a further dimension, especially in gauging disease activity throughout the body

7. Isotope scanning (e.g. gallium for nodes, technetium for liver/spleen/bone)—another adjunctive procedure of occasional value

Clinical features
1. Primarily affects young adults and middle-aged. Commoner in males
2. Commonest presentation—lymph node enlargement
   (i)   Cervical—in over 50% of patients
   (ii) Mediastinal—commonest in NS type. May obstruct superior vena cava, bronchus
   (iii) Other sites—nasopharyngeal, axillary, inguinal, pelvic and intra-abdominal
3. Nodes are firm, often discrete and mobile but may become matted
4. Constitutional ('B') symptoms, e.g. weight loss, fever and sweats (true Pel–Ebstein cyclical fever is unusual)—*usually* in association with widespread disease or a late feature
5. Alcohol induced pain at sites of disease, in a minority
6. Splenomegaly—frequent
7. Hepatomegaly—frequent. Jaundice may result from hepatic infiltration
8. HD can involve any tissue—the following are worth noting:
   (i)   Lung—diffuse or nodular, parenchymal or pleural (causing effusions)
   (ii) Bone—pain or pathological fracture (e.g. vertebral collapse)
   (iii) CNS—cord compression due to extradural mass or collapsed vertebrae. Non-specific—progressive leuco-encephalopathy
9. Infective complications—opportunistic infections (reflecting immunodeficiency)

Staging

Procedures
Determination of the extent of disease is essential for rational treatment. The procedures required are:
(i)   Clinical examination (including ENT assessment)
(ii) Imaging procedures—usually a combination, though whole-body CT scanning is now commonly used for baseline and follow-up assessments
(iii) Bone marrow trephine
(iv) Laparotomy (with splenectomy)—less commonly carried out because:
   a. Chemotherapy is usually effective in patients relapsing after initial radiotherapy
   b. Non-invasive investigations, particularly imaging, provide reasonably accurate information

Clinical staging system:
1. Stage I—involvement of a single lymph node region
   (LNR)/lymphoid structure (spleen, thymus, Waldeyer's ring) *or*
   single localised extralymphatic site (ELS)
2. Stage II—involvement of two or more LNR/lymphoid structures
   or one localised ELS plus one or more LNR, *same* side of
   diaphragm
   Note: Subscript added to indicate number of LNR (e.g. II$_3$)
3. Stage III—involvement of LNR/lymphoid structures on *both*
   sides of the diaphragm
   Note: 'E' subscript added for limited ELS involvement
4. Stage IV—Extensive diffuse/disseminated involvement of one or
   more ELS—liver, marrow, pleura, lung, bone, skin:
   A. Absence of qualifying B symptoms
   B. Presence of qualifying symptoms:
       (i)   Unexplained weight loss > 10% body weight over
              previous 6 months
       (ii)   Unexplained persistent/recurrent fever with temperatures
              > 38°C during previous month
       (iii) Recurrent drenching night sweats during previous
              months
     Criteria for bulk:
     (i)   Palpable nodes: node/nodal mass > 10 cm largest diameter
     (ii)   Abdominal nodes: as for palpable nodes, but assessed by
            CT, ultrasound, lymphography or MRI
     (iii) Mediastinal mass—maximum width ≥ one-third of internal
            transverse diameter of thorax (standardised PA chest X-ray)
     Note: 'X' subscript may be added to denote bulky disease
     Pathological stage (PS)—based on additional biopsy
   information, as from laparotomy, e.g. CSIII$_4$A; PSIII$_s$A (spleen
   involved).

Treatment
The objective is to induce complete remission (CR), i.e. no evidence
of disease clinically *and* on re-investigation. Choice of treatment is
linked to stage.

1. Radiotherapy
(i)   As first-line treatment for non-bulky disease of limited extent
       with good prognostic features (within categories IA and IIA)
(ii)   For residual disease following chemotherapy
(iii) To the site of previously bulky disease following
       chemotherapy
(iv)   To sites of localised recurrent disease

2. Chemotherapy
Now generally the first-line treatment apart from in the good
prognostic stages IA and IIA.
(i)   A well-tried combination is MOPP (mustine hydrochloride,

vincristine, procarbazine and prednisolone) given in courses
every 3–4 weeks
(ii) In an attempt to improve remission rates and long-term results,
multi-drug alternating combinations have been introduced, e.g.
MOPP-ABVD (adriamycin, bleomycin, vinblastine, dacarbazine)
and ChIVPP (chlorambucil, vinblastine, procarbazine,
prednisolone-PABIOE (prednisolone, adriamycin, bleomycin,
vincristine, etoposide)
(iii) Because of long-term toxicities—permanant infertility in men
and secondary malignancies (especially leukaemia,
AML)—the effectiveness of less toxic combinations, e.g. those
omitting alkylating agents and procarbazine, is being
investigated
(iv) Intensive chemotherapy (± radiotherapy) followed by
autologous bone marrow transplantation (ABMT or 'marrow
rescue')—an increasingly adopted approach for relapsed
disease or as 'consolidation' therapy in younger patients with
poor prognostic features

Prognosis
1. Localised early stage disease: very high CR rate with the great
majority apparently cured
2. More advanced disease: a CR rate of about 85% is the norm;
long-term disease-free survival only about 60%
3. The presence of poor prognostic features, e.g. bulky disease
or indices based on several prognostic factors, may be used
as the basis for selecting patients for more aggressive
therapy

NON HODGKIN'S LYMPHOMAS (NHL)

Aetiology
A variety of exogenous causes have been implicated (viruses,
radiation, toxic chemicals), as well as genetic factors. With a
few notable exceptions best regarded as of multifactorial
aetiology.

Pathology
1. The cell proliferations are heterogeneous, forming a
discontinuous spectrum of disorders, and there has been
disagreement and confusion in their classification
2. Broad groupings have been distinguished on the basis of the
associated clinical picture and response to treatment—hence
'low-grade' for histology which generally carries a better
prognosis than 'high-grade'. The rate of cell proliferation is
generally low in low-grade, high in high-grade NHL.

3. One relatively simple classification (based on the Kiel system) is:
   Follicular:
   (i)   centrocytic
   (ii) centroblastic-centrocytic
   Diffuse:
   (i)   lymphocytic—CLL may be included ⎫
   (ii) lymphoplasmacytoid   ⎬ Low-grade
   (iii) centrocytic   ⎪
   (iv) centroblastic-centrocytic   ⎭
   (v)   centroblastic   ⎫
   (vi) immunoblastic   ⎬ High-grade
   (vii) lymphoblastic   ⎪
   (viii) 'Burkitt-type' (small non-cleaved cell) ⎭
4. Because there are more than two sharply demarcated patterns
   of disease, alternative groupings have been introduced. The
   Working Formulation, a system intended to aid comparisons
   between different classifications, has three grades—low,
   intermediate and high (see Appendix)
5. Other approaches are closely linked to modes of treatment
   —the NCI scheme identifies 'indolent', 'aggressive' and 'very
   aggressive' (or leukaemia-like) NHL
6. Immunological techniques which detect cell surface antigens
   have led to a better understanding of lymphoid cell
   differentiation/transformation; sub-categories can be
   characterised by cluster differentiation (CD) antigen markers
   and the immunophenotype characterised as 'mature' or
   'immature'
7. While the majority of NHL are B-cell in origin, both immature
   and mature T-cell diseases occur with significant differences in
   clinical behaviour
8. Indices of cell proliferation are also aids to characterisation and
   carry prognostic significance
9. Tend to be associated with more extranodal disease than HD
10. The anatomical site may influence clinical behaviour:
    (i)   Localised extranodal, arising in the lymphoid tissue
          of various organs—e.g. gut, skin, thyroid, salivary
          glands
    (ii) Gut—may be localised ± regional nodal involvement,
          multifocal or diffuse
    (iii) Mediastinal—notably T-lymphoblastic in children and
          young adults, often with leukaemia-like picture
11. Varying degrees of immunosuppression. Paraproteins are
    sometimes produced

Haematology
1. Often normal as in HD. Rarely, diagnostic
2. Anaemia as in HD
3. Lymphocytes may be increased

4. Blood film:
   (i) 'Atypical' lymphocytes may be present
   (ii) Circulating malignant lymphoid cells—in 'spill-over' or leukaemic transformation
5. ESR/plasma viscosity—crude guide to disease activity
6. Bone marrow—infiltration in up to 30% of low-grade, less than 15% of high-grade types

Cytogenetics
Many abnormalities have been identified in patients with NHL. Specific associations include:
1. t(8; 14) (q24; q32) translocation—in some high-grade NHL, e.g. Burkitt type; HIV-associated
2. t(14; 18) (q32; q21) and deregulation of the B-cell oncogene, bcl-12—common in follicular lymphomas

Biochemistry
1. Serum lactic dehydrogenase (LDH) — not a specific marker but reflects proliferative activity; marked increases tend to be associated with poor prognosis
2. Serum beta-2-microglobulin (β_2m) levels also tend to increase with increasing tumour load and (like LDH) may be used as a prognostic indicator
3. Acute-phase reactants, e.g. C-reactive protein (CRP) may be increased in active NHL—non-specific changes (also reflected in ESR and plasma viscosity)
4. Various biochemical disturbances, e.g. of liver function tests, may occur with disease progression and compromised organ function

Imaging
Essentially as for HD.

Clinical features
1. Heterogeneous group of diseases with greater variety of clinical manifestations than HD
2. Childhood presentation (of diffuse, high-grade forms) is not uncommon but otherwise predominantly diseases of middle and later life. Commoner in males
3. Nodal presentation is less frequent than in HD
4. Splenomegaly and/or hepatomegaly are common
5. Extra-nodal sites, primary (20% of all NHL) or secondary, include: orbit, nasopharynx, tonsil, GI tract, skin and bone
6. Symptoms may relate to primary infiltration, e.g. proptosis, malignant skin ulcer
7. Constitutional 'B' symptoms are less prominent than in HD, though fever is a feature of extensive disease

8. CNS involvement—meningeal infiltration (as in ALL) especially with poor prognosis histology and in childhood (30%)

Staging

1. A similar system to that used in HD may be applied but is less valid. Within any given stage there may be considerable differences in the nature of the proliferation, the tumour cell load and prognosis
2. Alternative systems based on the number of extensively involved nodal sites and the number of extranodal sites have been put forward
3. Biochemical measurements, notably of LDH and β_2m, have also been used for patient stratification
4. Many other prognostic factors have been identified by multivariant analysis—age, performance status, Hb level, WBC/lymphocyte count, ESR/plasma viscosity, sodium, albumin, bone marrow, liver and CNS involvement. 'Prognostic indices' based on combinations of such parameters have been produced but there is no generally accepted system

Treatment

The approaches to treatment are fundamentally different for low- and high-grade NHL

Low-grade NHL

Failure to achieve complete remission (CR) does not necessarily mean that disease control will not be achieved over a long period. The principal therapeutic approaches are:

1. 'Watch and wait'—minimal disease in the least aggressive categories may remain stable and asymptomatic
2. Chemotherapy:
    (i) Single alkylating agent, e.g. chlorambucil, usually given intermittently—often effective in achieving remissions and disease control
    (ii) Corticosteroids—can be of value, e.g. in initial treatment, improving bone marrow function
    (iii) Combinations, e.g. COP (cyclophosphamide, vincristine, prednisolone) or, with addition of an anthracycline, such as hydroxydaunorubicin in CHOP—may be required for more aggressive disease
3. Radiotherapy—principally for localised disease or to the spleen, as part of overall strategy
4. Surgery—also has a role in the treatment of truly localised disease

High-grade NHL

Of crucial importance to achieve true CRs for prolonged disease-free survival.

1. Chemotherapy—multi-drug combinations, the most proven of which is still CHOP; more intensive approaches may be indicated in certain categories and autologous bone marrow transplant (ABMT or 'marrow rescue') allows potentially lethal chemotherapy ± radiotherapy to be given relatively safely
2. Radiotherapy—may be effective in localised disease but is more often given adjuvently as part of overall therapeutic strategy, e.g. to residual mediastinal disease or pre-ABMT
3. Surgery—limited role in truly localised disease

Note: Those NHL regarded as of 'intermediate grade' include categories which also require 'high-grade' treatment. The leukaemia-like high-grade NHL, notably T- and B-lymphoblastic, may be best treated with drug schedules as adopted for acute lymphoblastic leukaemia (see p.113)

Supportive measures
Patients with NHL are variously at risk of developing opportunistic infective complications because of associated immunodeficiencies and the effects of treatment. Measures which may be taken include:
1. Prophylaxis against specific infections, e.g. cotrimoxazole (for *Pneumocystis carinii*), acyclovir (for herpes virus group) and penicillin V in high-risk patients
2. Prompt institution of empiric antimicrobials for pyrexial episodes

Prognosis
Age and performance status, which are important prognostic factors, may influence the therapeutic approach and thereby outcome.

1. Low-grade NHL:
(i) Although partial remission and disease stability are the most that is achieved in the majority this is compatible with prolonged survival (>5 years in 75% of patients)
(ii) Appreciable differences between the various histologies (e.g. the more aggressive forms included in the 'intermediate grade' of the Working Formulation have intrinsically poorer outlook)
(iii) Transformation to high-grade disease is usually associated with rapid disease progression and poor response to treatment

2. High-grade NHL:
(i) Truly localised non-bulky disease—a very high complete remission (CR) rate and prolonged disease-free survival (DFS) in the great majority (80–90%)
(ii) More extensive and generalised disease—CR rates of the order of 75% are achieved with prolonged DFS in about 50% of

patients; intensive treatment with or without allograft/autograft in very aggressive NHL may improve overall results

(iii) Relapsed disease—'salvage' treatment, including intensive treatment with allograft/autograft, is resulting in 25% DFS

SPECIAL CATEGORIES

LYMPHOBLASTIC (LEUKAEMIA-LIKE) NHL

1. T-cell — derived from immature T cells of thymic origin:
   (i) Disease of children and young adults
   (ii) Closely related to acute T-cell lymphoblastic leukaemia (ALL)
   (iii) Pathology—large, blastic cells with scanty cytoplasm and indented or convoluted nuclei; positive for T-cell markers
   (iv) Clinically, mediastinal nodal enlargement is typical. Leukaemic manifestations are usually early. High risk of CNS involvement
   (v) Treatment—chemotherapy as for ALL with CNS prophylaxis
2. B cell:
   (i) rarer than T-cell type; in similar age group
   (ii) essentially identical to B-cell lymphoblastic leukaemia (ALL)
   (iii) Pathology—FAB L_3-type morphology (see Table 14.1, p.110); high tumour growth fraction; association with t(8;14) translocation
   (iv) Clinically—tendency to bulky disease, e.g. intra-abdominal and CNS involvement
   (v) Treatment—intensive, as for ALL; poor prognosis

BURKITT'S LYMPHOMA (B-CELL MALIGNANCY)

1. First observed by Burkitt in African children in 1957
2. Epstein–Barr virus (EBV) implicated; immunosuppressive effects of endemic malaria a risk factor
3. Histopathology—uniform cytology of malignant B lymphoid cells with cytoplasmic basophilia; scattered macrophages produce a 'starry sky' effect
4. Cytogenetics—characteristic t(8;14) translocation
5. Clinical features—rapidly progressive disease with predisposition to extranodal involvement, e.g. intra-abdominal sites, facial bones, CNS (50%)
6. Treatment—usually a good initial response to chemotherapy (80% remission rate) but CNS disease carries poor prognosis

ADULT T-CELL LEUKAEMIA/LYMPHOMA (ATL)

As with Burkitt's lymphoma, of considerable interest because of the viral connection.

1. Seen in various parts of Japan and the West Indies
2. Human lymphotropic virus type I (HTLV-1) implicated; transmitted:
   (i)   Transplacentally or via breast feeding
   (ii) Heterosexual transmission
   (iii) By blood transfusion
3. The malignant cells are activated peripheral T cells; circulating abnormal lymphoid cells often detected
4. Clinical features—generalised lymphadenopathy, hepatosplenomegaly and lytic bone lesions with hypercalcaemia
5. Usual aggressive course; may respond to combination chemotherapy

HIV-ASSOCIATED LYMPHOMA

There is an increased incidence of diffuse NHL in patients with HIV disease, a reflection of the associated immunosuppression and not directly caused by the virus.
1. Usually high-grade and of B-cell origin (probably EBV/CMV stimulated)
2. High incidence of extranodal and primary brain disease
3. May show response to combination chemotherapy but often relapses early—of poor prognosis

PERIPHERAL T CELL NHL

1. Derived from mature post-thymic T cells
2. Comprise about 20% diffuse NHL (mycosis fungoides excluded)
3. Morphologically and immunologically diverse group
4. A simple classification based on principal cell features:
   (i)   atypical lymphocytic (low grade)
   (ii) mixed cell (intermediate grade)
   (iii) large cell (high grade)
5. Clinical features: various but systemic ('B') symptoms, generalised lymphadenopathy and stage III/IV disease common
6. Treatment essentially as for B-cell NHL; prognosis probably less good than B-cell equivalents

MYCOSIS FUNGOIDES (T-CELL MALIGNANCY)

Primarily a skin lymphoma, it may become generalised (with fever, weight loss, lymphadenopathy and hepatosplenomegaly) and may develop into the Sézary syndrome.

SÉZARY SYNDROME (T-CELL MALIGNANCY)

Closely related to mycosis fungoides. The pathognomonic cell, atypical lymphoid with cerebriform nucleus, is found in blood, skin and lymph nodes of patients with erythroderma.

PRIMARY GUT LYMPHOMAS

Represent 1–2% of all gastrointestinal malignancies.
  In addition to primary lesions of the previously described principal NHL, there are forms peculiar to the gut:
1. B-cell:
     (i)   Lymphomas, typically low-grade, arising in mucosa-associated lymphoid tissue (MALTomas), but with pleomorphic high-grade equivalent (possibly a transformation from low-grade)
     (ii)   Immunoproliferative disease of small intestine (or α chain disease, see p.87)
     (iii) Multiple lymphomatous polyposis—polypoid accumulation of malignant centrocytes; high frequency of dissemination outside GI tract
     (iv)   Burkitt-like
2. T-cell:
     Enteropathy-associated T-cell lymphoma (EATL)—pleomorphic large cell proliferation often associated with villous atrophy; may be history of preceding coeliac disease and the clinical presentation is commonly that of malabsorption

ANGIOIMMUNOBLASTIC LYMPHADENOPATHY

1. Aberrant T-cell disorders in which there are varying degrees of dysplasia, including a premalignant state; clonality can be demonstrated in about 60% of cases. May be triggered by a hypersensitivity reaction
2. Histopathology—proliferation of small vessels with polymorphic cellular reaction/proliferation
3. Haematology—haemolytic anaemia (Coombs-positive) frequent
4. Immunology—polyclonal hyperglobulinaemia
5. Clinical features—systemic ('B') symptoms with generalised lymphadenopathy and hepatosplenomegaly. Rashes are common
6. Course and prognosis—unpredictable but often fatal. No specific therapy

HISTIOCYTIC MEDULLARY RETICULOSIS

1. Pathology—T-cell disease but with cytokine-induced histiocytic (macrophage) reactive changes (including erythrophagocytosis)
2. Haematology:
     (i)   Pancytopenia usual
     (ii)   Blood film—abnormal mononuclear cells

(iii) Bone marrow—abnormal macrophages, phagocytosing red cells, platelets etc.
3. Biochemistry—serum lysozyme may be increased (reflecting macrophage activity)
4. Clinical features—persistent or recurrent pyrexia, malaise and weight loss; hepatosplenomegaly ± lymphadenopathy
5. Treatment—combination chemotherapy, e.g. CHOP, may induce response and remission

NON-MALIGNANT LYMPHOPROLIFERATIVE DISEASES
INFECTIOUS MONONUCLEOSIS

Has been called a 'self-limiting' neoplasm but should be distinguished from a malignant process.

Pathogenesis
1. Epstein-Barr virus (EBV) enters lymphoid system via pharyngeal tissue, infects/transforms B cells which, in turn, induce a florid cytotoxic T-cell response
2. Atypical lymphocytic infiltration, chiefly of reticuloendothelial system (differentiation from lymphoma may be difficult)
3. The abnormal cells are larger than normal lymphocytes with abundant basophilic cytoplasm, often vacuolated (similar to 'transformed' lymphocytes seen in vitro)

Haematology
1. Anaemia—not usually a feature but secondary/haemolytic anaemia may occur
2. Mild to moderate lymphocytosis usual (rarely > 30 × 10^9/l)
3. Platelets—slight decrease common. Rarely, marked thrombocytopenia
4. Blood film—atypical lymphocytes, increasing during the clinical illness

Serology
1. Heterophile (anti-sheep/horse) antibodies (IgM)—absorbable by beef erythroblasts but not guinea-pig kidney (Paul–Bunnell test)
2. A variety of IgM antibodies may be produced; some may act as cold agglutinins
3. Antibody titre reaches peak in second or third week

Biochemistry
1. Abnormal liver function tests—SGOT, γGT and alkaline phosphatase frequently increased; occasionally, severe derangement
2. Abnormal protein pattern with increased IgM

Clinical features
1. Disease predominantly of older children and young adults—common in institutions, e.g. hospitals
2. Presentation—malaise, fever, headache, anorexia, sore throat (80%), lymph node enlargement (usually cervical)
3. Pyrexia—variable, usually moderate
4. Lymph nodes moderately enlarged, discrete and often tender
5. Splenomegaly (about 50%); hepatomegaly (about 20%)
6. Pharyngeal mucosal injection common (± exudate)

Complications
1. Hepato-cellular damage with jaundice (5%)
2. Pathological blood loss due to thrombocytopenia (rare)

Treatment
No specific therapy. Supportive in severe cases.

Prognosis
In the vast majority of cases, there is complete resolution of symptoms and physical signs within several weeks.

TRUE HISTIOCYTIC PROLIFERATIVE DISORDERS

Although these have clinical features in common with NHL, i.e. lymphoproliferative disease, the malignant cells have the immunological markers of the monocyte/macrophage series. Management as for high-grade NHL.

MISCELLANEOUS HISTIOCYTIC DISEASES

These include sinus histiocytosis (benign but associated with massive lymphadenopathy) and histiocytosis X.

IMMUNOPROLIFERATIVE DISORDERS

There is a spectrum of conditions from benign to malignant, involving potentially immunoglobulin-producing lymphoid cells (B cells) which may be distinguished within the lymphoproliferative disorders.

IMMUNOGLOBULINS

1. Differ from all other proteins in variability, diversity, genetic control and in having antibody specificity
2. Consist of two heavy and two light polypeptide chains
3. Exist in five classes—IgG, IgA, IgM, IgD and IgE
4. Have corresponding heavy chains: γ, α, μ, δ and ϵ

5. Have one of two light chains—kappa (κ) and lambda (λ)
6. Have molecular weight 150 000 to 200 000 *except* IgM (900 000)
7. Are monoclonal when they are produced by cells derived from a single clone (i.e. from a single tumour stem cell)
8. When monoclonal ('paraprotein') are true to type and only a single light chain type can be detected
9. When polyclonal, as in the normal antibody reaction to infection, represent a broad spectrum of globulins

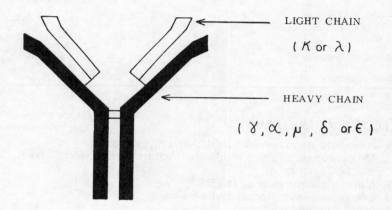

LIGHT CHAIN

$(K \text{ or } \lambda)$

HEAVY CHAIN

$(\gamma, \alpha, \mu, \delta \text{ or } \epsilon)$

Fig. 9.2   Basic structure of immunoglobulin

MONOCLONAL GAMMOPATHIES OR PARAPROTEINAEMIAS

May be due to:
1. Monoclonal gammopathies of undetermined significance (MGUS)
2. Equivocal myeloma   } sub-types as shown in Table 9.1
3. Myelomatosis
4. Macroglobulinaemia (IgM)

MGUS

Affects 1–3% population; asymptomatic. Features include:
1. Monoclonal gammopathy, remaining static over long periods
2. Monoclonal (M)—component level of less than 25g/l with no immune paresis, and BJ level of < 1 g/24 hours
3. Marrow plasma cells < 10%
4. Bone lesions absent
5. β_2 microglobulin < 2 mg/l
6. Haematology and renal function normal

7. Requires regular follow-up, as up to 30% progress to myeloma within 10 years. Treatment not required

Table 9.1. Sub-types of myelomatosis (based on 1600 patients from MRC Myeloma Trials I–IV)

Type	%
IgG	55
A	27
D	1.5
M	0.2
Bence-Jones only	15
Non-secretory	1

'EQUIVOCAL' MYELOMA

Intermediate stage between MGUS and myeloma:
1. M-component ≥ 25 g/l $\pm$ moderate immune paresis, and BJ level of < 1 g/24 hours
2. Marrow plasma cells up to 25%
3. One or less asymptomatic lytic lesion
4. β_2 microglobulin < 4 mg/l
5. Haematology and renal function normal
6. No evidence of progressive myeloma
7. Requires regular follow-up; treatment not required

MYELOMATOSIS (MULTIPLE MYELOMA)

Pathology
1. Neoplastic proliferation of plasma cells:
    (i)   Diffuse or patchy replacement of normal bone marrow tissue with variable interference with normal haematopoiesis
    (ii) Destruction of medullary and cortical bone, causing lytic lesions and sometimes pathological fractures
    (iii) Infiltration of other body tissues
2. Production of paraprotein (monoclonal gammopathy) and/or light chain moiety:
    (i)   Impaired production of normal immunoglobulins, e.g. in antibody formation
    (ii) Interference with renal function, in particular by Bence-Jones (light chain) proteinuria
    (iii) Interference with clotting factors and platelet function

(iv) Increased plasma viscosity (depending on type and quantity of paraprotein)
3. Amyloidosis (approximately 10%)—distribution as in primary amyloid disease (e.g. skin, heart, gastrointestinal tract)

Haematology
1. Anaemia, usually normochromic, normocytic
2. Neutropenia and thrombocytopenia, usually only in later stages
3. Blood film —marked rouleaux formation and increased bluish background staining (secondary to protein changes). Plasma cells may be seen (15%) and a leucoerythroblastic picture may develop (10%)
4. ESR—usually very high (except in Bence-Jones myelomatosis)
5. Bone marrow—typically infiltrated with $\geq$ 20–30% plasma cells (the morphology of which varies from normal to immature)
   Note:
   (i)   Increases of up to about 10% plasma cells may be 'reactive' (e.g. in chronic inflammation)
   (ii) Marrow involvement may be patchy (i.e. false negatives possible); trephine biopsy often more representative
6. Increased plasma viscosity—markedly so in some patients, notably those with polymerising IgA paraproteinaemia
7. Defective clotting function (variable)
8. cALLA positivity of plasma cells and peripheral blood B lymphocytes associated with poor prognosis

Biochemistry

1. Serum
(i)   Increased total protein due to raised globulin
(ii)   Reduced albumin (frequent)
(iii) Homogeneous band of protein on serum electrophoresis ('M' band)
(iv)   Paraprotein (and light chain class) identified by immunoelectrophoresis, e.g. IgG kappa
(v)   Immunoparesis—reduced levels of the normal immunoglobulins
(vi)   Increased blood urea and serum creatinine (evidence of severe renal impairment often late)
(vii) Increased serum calcium—often late (usually due to a combination of increased bone resorption and renal functional impairment)
(viii) Increased β_2 microglobulin (partly due to impaired renal clearance)
(ix)   Increased LDH

2. Urine
(i)   Bence-Jones (light chain) proteinuria—in vitro, flocculation

occurs at 45–60°C, disappears on boiling (variable)
Immunoelectrophoresis or isoelectric focusing confirms
(ii) Albuminuria (common)
(iii) Tubulo-proteinuria (reflecting tubular damage)

Clinical features
1. Maximum incidence 50–70 years of age. Commoner in males
2. Bone destruction—osteoporosis, and 'punched-out' lytic lesions due to the production of 'osteoclast activating factors' (IL_1, TNF_α and β, IL_6)
   (i)   Bony aches and pains and tenderness, especially in the back and ribs
   (ii) Spontaneous or post-traumatic pathological fractures, e.g. ribs and spine (vertebral collapse)
   (iii) Tumour formation, e.g. ribs. Rarely an isolated lesion (solitary plasmacytoma)
3. Sequelae of marrow replacement—anaemia, cytopenias
4. Sequelae of immunoparesis—infections
5. Neurological symptoms due to :
   (i)   Pressure of myeloma tissue, e.g. on spinal cord/nerve roots
   (ii) Bone destruction, e.g. vertebral collapse, which may cause sudden paraplegia
   (iii) Amyloidosis, e.g. peripheral neuropathy
6. Uraemia—usually late, though some patients present with renal failure
7. Features of hypercalcaemia—nausea, thirst, constipation, drowsiness
8. Hyperviscosity syndrome—unusual (but see macro-globulinaemia, p.85)
9. Hepatomegaly (40%), splenomegaly (10%). Lymphadenopathy is rare
10. Easy bruising. Haemorrhages (e.g. fundal) due to thrombocytopenia or defective platelet function secondary to paraprotein coating and interference with clotting cascade

Staging
Symptoms appear when the myeloma cell burden is between 2×10^{11} and 4×10^{12} cells. There is broad correlation between certain clinical criteria and tumour mass—high tumour mass is likely with one or all of the following:
1. Marked anaemia
2. Hypercalcaemia
3. Extensive lytic bone lesions
4. IgG > 70 g/l, IgA > 50 g/l and/or urine light chain excretion > 12 g/24 hours

Treatment
1. Basic concepts:
    (i)   Induction of complete remission is rarely achieved
    (ii) In responding patients paraprotein levels usually decrease
          to a particular level and then stabilise in 'plateau', which
          often continues for prolonged periods whether or not
          treatment is continued
    (iii) The clinical criteria of response are difficult to categorise;
          e.g. relief of bone pain may be of prime importance to the
          patient
    (iv) Response to therapy in terms of paraprotein—reduction to
          below 25% of original serum level is significant. Treat for 6
          months after achieving plateau
2. Chemotherapy:
    (i)   Alkylating agents—melphalan and cyclophosphamide are
          both effective agents in inducing remissions and prolonging
          survival
    (ii) Corticosteroids—prednisolone can enhance alkylating agent
          therapy initially, though longer-term benefits dubious;
          intermediate-dose pulsed prednisolone may also be
          effective in advanced disease inducing partial remissions
          with clinical and biochemical responses
    (iii) Other agents, e.g. anthracyclines, nitrosoureas and vinca
          alkaloids, produce responses, notably in combination
          therapy, e.g. ABCM, VAD
    (iv) α-interferons—preliminary studies suggest that
          maintenance treatment prolongs duration of plateau phase
          remission
    (v)   2-deoxycoformicin, an adenosine deaminase inhibitor, may
          be effective in advanced myeloma. Contraindicated in
          presence of uraemia
    (vi) High-dose chemotherapy, e.g. melphalan in combination
          with TBI and autologous bone marrow rescue—a more
          'aggressive' approach which may produce good remissions
          and, possibly, prolonged survival
    (vii) Duration of therapy depends on evidence of continuing
          response; increased risk of drug resistance and leukaemic
          transformation with long-term chemotherapy—patients in
          continuing plateau phase are not usually given treatment,
          though maintenance with α-interferon may prove
          beneficial
3. Radiotherapy:
    (i)   To painful local lesions to relieve pain
    (ii) To vertebrae to prevent further collapse (not of certain
          value)
    (iii) To extradural deposits to prevent spinal cord compression
4. Treatment of hypercalcaemia:
    (i)   Vigorous rehydration—often produces an immediate effect

with improvement in renal function (at least 3 litres fluid/24 hours input recommended)
  (ii) Hypocalcaemic agents, e.g. diphosphonates, mithramycin, high dose corticosteroids and calcitonin
  (iii) Specific chemotherapy as above
  (iv) Mobilisation (bed rest aggravates osteolysis)
5. Supportive:
  (i)   Rehydration and maintenance of optimal hydration
  (ii) Prompt treatment of infections
  (iii) Plasmapheresis for hyperviscosity (see macro-globulinaemia)
  (iv) Dialysis for renal failure

Table 9.2.   Prognostic features in myelomatosis

	Good	Bad
Haemoglobin	>10 g/dl	<7.5 g/dl
Urea	<8 mmol/l	>10 mmol/l
Albumin	<30 g/l	<30 g/l
Calcium	<2.5 µmol/l	>2.5 µmol/l
β_2 microglobulin	<4 mg/l	>6 mg/l
cALLA (CD10)	Negative	Positive
Plasma cell labelling index (3_H thymidine/bromodeoxyuridine)	Low	High
Chromosomal abnormalities	Absent	Present

Prognosis
1. Untreated—median survival 9–12 months
2. Treated with current regimens—median survival 2 years (though patients presenting with poor prognostic features, especially severe renal impairment, have a median survival of about 2 months)
3. Intensive combination regimens ± ABMT may improve survival rates (subject of therapeutic studies)

MACROGLOBULINAEMIA

IgM paraprotein may be associated with:
1. Malignant disease:
  (i)   Non-Hodgkin's lymphoma
  (ii) Waldenström's macroglobulinaemia
  (iii) IgM myelomatosis (rare)
  (iv) Chronic lymphocytic leukaemia (rare association)

2. Benign disorders:
   (i)   Cold haemagglutinin disease
   (ii) Autoimmune disease (e.g. rheumatoid arthritis)

WALDENSTRÖM'S MACROGLOBULINAEMIA

Pathology
1. Proliferation of lymphocytes, plasmacytoid lymphocytes and plasma cells
2. Infiltration of bone marrow, lymph nodes, liver, spleen and other tissues
3. Lymph node architecture largely preserved
4. IgM paraproteinaemia:
   (i)   Tendency to increased blood viscosity
   (ii) Interference with platelet function and clotting factors

Haematology
1. Peripheral blood—essentially as for myelomatosis
2. Markedly increased plasma viscosity—common, due to IgM pentamers
3. Bone marrow—classically, an excess of plasmacytoid lymphocytes

Biochemistry
1. Paraprotein of IgM type identified by immunoelectrophoresis
2. Bence-Jones proteinuria in 10%

Clinical features
1. Usually presents in patients aged 50–70. Commoner in males
2. Insidious onset is usual
3. Symptoms and signs often relate to the hyperviscosity syndrome:
   (i)   Tiredness, loss of appetite, weight and energy
   (ii) Increasing visual disturbances—due to venous engorgement, haemorrhages and, sometimes, papilloedema
   (iii) Neurological changes—central and/or peripheral, focal and/or generalised
   (iv) Haemorrhagic tendency—bruising, bleeding
4. Hepatosplenomegaly and lymphadenopathy occur (not usually marked)

Treatment
1. Chemotherapy—chlorambucil may be very effective though responses may not be seen for several months (corticosteroids are often of additional value initially)
2. Plasmapheresis—often crucial initially when there is marked hyperviscosity and before chemotherapy is effective. Reduces

viscosity rapidly because IgM paraprotein is predominantly intravascular

Prognosis
Although the course of disease may be relatively benign, as many as 50% of patients are dead at 5 years. There is an increased risk of development of second malignancies.

CRYOGLOBULINAEMIA

Cryoglobulins have the property of precipitation or gel formation at low temperatures (below 37°C). May or may not be monoclonal.

Classification
Three main types of cryoglobulins can be distinguished:
1. Type I—isolated monoclonal paraproteins or light chains
2. Type II—mixed cryoglobulins, immunoglobulins ± monoclonal component
3. Type III—mixed polyclonal immunoglobulins of one or more class, sometimes including non-immunoglobulin molecules, e.g. complement

Associations
1. Myelomatosis—may be IgG, IgA, IgM or light chain (Type I)
2. Waldenström's macroglobulinaemia (Type I)
3. Malignant lymphoma, nearly always non-Hodgkin's (usually Type II)
4. Connective-tissue disease, e.g. SLE (Type III)
5. Infections (Type III)

Clinical features
1. Circulatory abnormalities induced by cold; in severe cases, gangrene. Severity of symptoms depends on thermal range of cryoglobulin
2. Hyperviscosity syndrome

Treatment
Of the underlying disease.

HEAVY CHAIN DISEASE

Production of monoclonal protein heavy chain fragments. These are *rare* diseases:

1. Gamma (γ) chain disease (Franklin's disease)
(i) Lymph nodes and marrow show plasmacytic/histiocytic infiltration
(ii) Serum and urine contain the heavy chain fragment (Fc portion)

(iii) Clinical picture—that of malignant lymphoma, predominantly in middle-aged/elderly males
(iv) Prognosis—poor, with survival usually less than 1 year; resistant to therapy

2. Alpha (α) chain disease (immunoproliferative disease of small intestine)

(i) Malignant proliferation of IgA-secreting B lymphoid cells with infiltration of small bowel mucosa by plasma cells and immunoblasts
(ii) Serum, urine and jejunal fluid contain the heavy chain fragment
(iii) Clinical picture—of malabsorption, predominantly in children or young adults (especially of Mediterranean stock)
(iv) Prognosis—poor; frequently terminates in death from wasting syndrome or transformation to malignant plasmacytoma

3. Mu (μ) chain disease

Very rare indeed; may occur in chronic lymphocytic leukaemia.

FURTHER ADVANCED READING

Aisenberg A C 1991 Malignant lymphoma. Biology, Natural History and Treatment. Lea and Febiger, Philadelphia

Delamore I W (ed) 1986 Multiple myeloma and other paraproteinaemias. Churchill Livingstone, Edinburgh

Durie E G M 1986 Plasma cell disorders. In: Hoffbrand A V (ed) Recent advances in haematology 5. Churchill Livingstone, Edinburgh, pp 305–327

McElwain T J, Lister T A (eds) 1987 The lymphomas. Clinical Haematology vol. 1:1. Baillière Tindall, London

Selby P J, McElwain T J (eds) 1987 Hodgkin's disease. Blackwell Scientific Publications, Oxford

10. Chronic myeloproliferative disorders

Basic features

1. Autonomous proliferation of one or more of the haemopoietic cell lines—erythroid, granulocytic, megakaryocytic
2. Marrow fibrosis, varying from negligible to marked—the dominant feature in myelofibrosis
3. Haematopoiesis in extramedullary sites may occur in any of these disorders

POLYCYTHAEMIA RUBRA VERA (PRV)

Aetiology

Clonal disorder, with erythroid progenitors showing hypersensitivity to erythropoietin stimulus. *Not* due to hypoxia, renal disease, etc. (see secondary polycythaemia, p.98).

Pathology

1. Orderly overproduction of erythrocytes and often granulocytes and platelets by the bone marrow
2. Absolute increase in red cell mass—blood volume increased
3. Increased viscosity due to increased haematocrit—one factor underlying a thrombotic tendency
4. Vascular engorgement—one factor underlying a haemorrhagic tendency
5. Extramedullary haematopoiesis may be present, notably in liver and spleen
6. Portal hypertension may result from:
   (i)   Pre-sinusoidal thrombosis
   (ii) Sinusoidal thrombosis
   (iii) High portal blood flow
   (iv) Post-sinusoidal thrombosis (Budd–Chiari syndrome)

Haematology

1. Hb, RBC and PCV increased
2. Leucocytosis, due to neutrophilia (>50% of patients)
3. Thrombocytosis—platelets occasionally $> 1000 \times 10^9$/l. Platelet aggregation (e.g. to ADP) impaired ± other qualitative defects

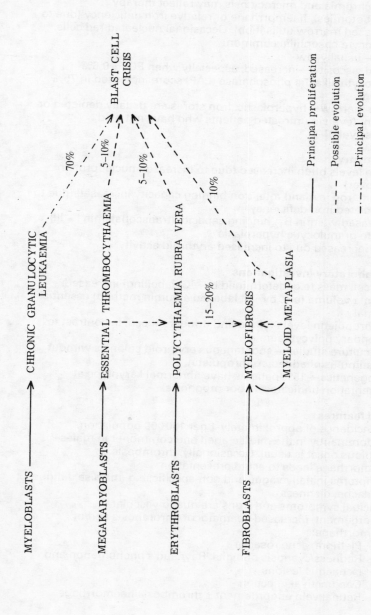

Fig. 10.1 Interrelationships between the myeloproliferative diseases

4. Blood film—red cells initially normochromic and normocytic—hypochromia and microcytosis may reflect therapy (phlebotomies), haemorrhage or relative iron deficiency (due to increased marrow utilisation). Occasional nucleated red cells. Leucocyte basophilia common.
5. ESR—usually low
6. Blood viscosity—increased, especially when PCV >0.6%
7. Leucocyte alkaline phosphatase (LAP) score increased in 75% patients
8. Bone marrow—hyperplastic. Iron stores are usually depleted or absent (even in untreated patients who have not bled excessively)

Biochemistry
1. Urate levels often increased (due to increased nucleoprotein turnover)
2. Serum iron low and total iron binding capacity increased (due to associated iron deficiency)
3. Increased vitamin B_{12} binding capacity (transcobalamin I + III) due to granulocytic hyperplasia
4. LDH increased due to increased erythroid activity

Other laboratory investigations
1. Red cell mass (e.g. determined by ^{51}Cr labelling) increased.
2. Plasma volume (e.g. by ^{125}I labelled albumin method) essentially normal
3. Erythropoietin levels (blood and urine) reduced, in contrast to secondary polycythaemia
4. Cell culture studies—spontaneous erythroid colonies without the stimulus of added erythropoietin
5. Cytogenetics—15% patients have abnormal karyotype at presentation (indicates a poor prognosis)

Clinical features
1. An incidence of approximately 1 per 100 000 population. Predominantly in the middle-aged and commoner in males
2. Insidious onset is usual. Occasionally, thrombosis or haemorrhage leads to acute presentation
3. Symptoms initially vague and non-specific, e.g. malaise, fatigue, headache, dizziness
4. Principal symptoms and signs are due to vascular engorgement, increased haematocrit, thrombosis and/or haemorrhage:
   (i) Plethora, acne rosacea
   (ii) Redness/cyanosis of digits. Raynaud's phenomenon and ischaemic lesions
   (iii) Conjunctival injection
   (iv) Retinal vein engorgement ± thrombosis/haemorrhage

(v) Hypertension (about 50% of patients). Occasionally myocardial infarction

(vi) Cerebrovascular accidents (thrombosis/haemorrhage, transient ischaemic attacks)

(vii) Intra-abdominal thrombosis—splenic, mesenteric. Budd–Chiari syndrome

(viii) Bleeding at various sites, e.g. skin, GI tract

5. Splenomegaly (>60% of patients) and often, hepatomegaly
6. Pruritus—common (20—25%), especially following a hot bath (related to basophilia and excessive histamine production ± associated iron deficiency)
7. Peptic ulceration/gastritis (up to 30% of patients)
8. Portal hypertension—another cause of GI haemorrhage
9. Gout (5%)

Differential diagnosis—secondary polycythaemia (see p.98) must be excluded.

Treatment

1. Venesection—rapid symptomatic relief and satisfactory control of mild disease. Aim is to keep PCV <0.45. Higher incidence of thrombotic complications than in ^{32}P or cytotoxic therapy
2. Radio-active phosphorus (^{32}P) at dose of 3–5 mCi i.v.— myelosuppression usually within 4–6 weeks (maximum effect by 12 weeks). Treatment of choice for elderly patients
3. Chemotherapy—alternative myelosuppressive therapy, requiring more supervision than ^{32}P. Alkylating agents associated with an increased risk of leukaemic transformation. Hydroxyurea (an antimetabolite) is safer, and is the preferred treatment in young patients not controlled by venesection

Course and prognosis

1. Untreated patients—death usually due to thrombosis or haemorrhage. Median survival about 5 years
2. Treated patients (with stable counts)—median survival about 13 years
3. The disease may 'evolve' with development of:
   (i) Clinically significant myeloid metaplasia and myelofibrosis (15–20%)
   (ii) Hypersplenism
   (iii) Leukaemic transformation in 5–10% (disease/treatment-related)
   (iv) Myelodysplasia (minority of patients)

PRIMARY (ESSENTIAL/IDIOPATHIC) THROMBOCYTHAEMIA (THROMBOCYTOSIS)

Definition

Increased platelet production due to a clonal myeloproliferative disorder and *not* reactive to, e.g. an inflammatory process, malignancy or haemorrhage. Most commonly seen in patients >50 years of age.

Haematology
1. Hb and PCV usually normal
2. Platelets—increased, often > 1000 × 10^9/l. Aggregation in vitro often impaired
3. Blood film—large and/or atypical platelets and sometimes megakaryocyte fragments
4. Bone marrow—megakaryocytes increased and frequently clumped; sheets of aggregated platelets commonly seen. Reticulin increased but marrow fibrosis not a feature

Clinical features
1. Splenomegaly (30–50% patients)
2. Pathological haemorrhages
3. Thromboembolic episodes:
   (i)   microvascular due to platelet aggregates, e.g. amaurosis fugax, digital skin ischaemia
   (ii) large-vessel disease, e.g. coronary thrombosis

Treatment
1. Antiplatelet drugs—e.g. aspirin—reduce platelet aggregation in vivo, but do not affect platelet count
2. ^{32}P—effective control may be achieved with relatively little therapy
3. Cytotoxic agents—alternative myelosuppression. Antimetabolites safer than alkylating agents, but not always effective
4. α-interferon—clinical trials in progress
5. Platelet apheresis—useful means of rapidly reducing platelet count in emergency situations. Transfusion of normally functioning platelets may then be necessary to control haemorrhage

Course and prognosis
1. The probability of death from haemorrhage/thromboembolism is reduced if platelet counts are well controlled by treatment (median survival 8–10 years)
2. A more florid myeloproliferative disease, and ultimately blast cell transformation, may supervene

MYELOID METAPLASIA AND MYELOFIBROSIS

Pathology
1. Clonal disorder, arising de novo, or as end-stage of other myeloproliferative disorders

2. Extramedullary haematopoiesis, especially in spleen and liver—the principal feature in myeloid metaplasia
3. Hypersplenism—the cause of marked increase in plasma volume
4. Ineffective erythropoiesis
5. Varying degrees of fibrosis in the marrow—hence the terms myelofibrosis if marked and osteosclerosis when there is secondary ossification. Platelet-derived growth factor (PDGF) and platelet factor 4 production may stimulate fibroblast proliferation.

Haematology
1. Anaemia, normochromic, normocytic
2. WBC—moderate increase usual but may be normal or reduced
3. Platelets—counts may be normal, increased or reduced (in the late stage)
4. Blood film—typically, leuco-erythroblastic:
   (i) Marked anisocytosis and poikilocytosis with tear-shaped red cells. Variable numbers of nucleated red cells
   (ii) Left shift in myeloid series—myelocytes and metamyelocytes present with occasional myeloblasts. LAP score usually increased
   (iii) Giant/atypical platelets often seen
5. Bone marrow—hyperplastic or variably hypoplastic with fibrosis. A 'dry-tap' is common; trephine biopsy shows the degree of fibrosis/ossification
6. Folate levels—reduced in about one-third of patients (a reflection of increased and ineffective erythropoiesis)
7. Isotopic studies—provide quantitative confirmation of:
   (i) Expanded plasma volume
   (ii) Splenic sequestration of red cells
   (iii) Extramedullary and medullary erythropoiesis (by ferrokinetic studies)

Biochemistry
1. Plasma urate levels—often increased
2. Bilirubin level—increases reflect the ineffective erythropoiesis
3. LDH—increased due to increased erythroid activity

Radiology
Increased bone density may be apparent.

Clinical features
1. Occurs predominantly in late middle and old age
2. Usually insidious in onset with the development of anaemia or increasing splenomegaly
3. Pathological haemorrhage—occasional (< 10%)
4. Bone pain—occasional

5. Systemic symptoms, e.g. fever, weight loss—usually late features
6. Splenomegaly may be massive. Hepatomegaly is usually moderate

Treatment
1. Supportive:
   (i)   Blood transfusion as required
   (ii) Folic acid supplements
   (iii) Allopurinol (to prevent gout)
2. Cytotoxic drugs—e.g. busulphan/hydroxyurea for more florid cases, to reduce spleen size, relieve pain and ameliorate systemic symptoms
3. Splenic irradiation—of temporary benefit. May relieve splenic pain and, by reducing spleen size, may improve Hb and PCV by reducing splenic RBC pool and plasma volume. FBC must be closely monitored
4. Splenectomy:
   (i)   Ideally, decision should be preceded by isotopic studies to assess erythropoietic capacity and plasma volume
   (ii) Of some value for splenic pain, marked hypersplenism, increasing transfusion requirements and portal hypertension
   (iii) Carries considerable operative risk; platelets may be greatly increased postoperatively (thromboembolic risk). Subsequent increased risk of life-threatening infection
   (iv) Probably best carried out early in the course of disease, if at all

Course and prognosis
1. Usually slowly progressive
2. Anaemia may be severe and demand repeated blood transfusions
3. Cardiovascular, haemorrhagic and infective complications may be fatal
4. Blast cell transformation occurs in about 10% of patients
5. Median survival, assuming careful management, about 5 years

MALIGNANT (ACUTE) MYELOFIBROSIS

1. Acute onset of anaemia, neutropenia and thrombocytopenia
2. Peripheral blood film—leuco-erythroblastic change with small numbers of circulating blasts
3. No evidence of gross hepatosplenomegaly
4. Seen in association with acute megakaryoblastic leukaemia (AML,M_7) and, occasionally, with lymphoma
5. Very poor prognosis

CHRONIC MYELOID (GRANULOCYTIC) LEUKAEMIA

Pathology
1. Development of malignant clone from pluripotent stem cell
2. Granulocytic hyperplasia in bone marrow with variable maturation defect
3. Predominance of cells of the granulocyte series at all stages of maturation in bone marrow (reflected in peripheral blood) during chronic phase, terminating with acute blastic transformation
4. Extramedullary haematopoiesis
5. Characteristic chromosomal abnormality (in 90% of patients) is the Philadelphia (Ph) chromosome (an abnormally short chromosome 22) due to reciprocal translocation t(9,22). Results in alignment of ABL oncogene (from chromosome 9) with breakpoint cluster region (BCR) of chromosome 22—the product of BCR-ABL is P210, with tyrosine kinase activity which presumably alters stem-cell kinetics
6. CGL without Ph chromosome has a number of different features (see p.97)

Haematology
1. Anaemia, usually normochromic, normocytic—increasingly severe with progressive disease
2. WBC—marked leucocytosis, typically $100–300 \times 10^9/l$, due to granulocytosis
3. Platelets—may be increased initially but often reduced as the disease progresses
4. Blood film:
   (i) Immature granulocytes, especially myelocytes (>25%)
   (ii) Increase in basophils
   (iii) LAP score reduced; an increase heralds acute blastic transformation
   (iv) Atypical platelets
5. Bone marrow—hypercellular with predominance of myeloid series, especially myelocytes. Ph chromosome present

Biochemistry
1. Plasma urate levels increased ⎫
2. LDH increased ⎬ reflecting high cell nucleoprotein turnover
3. Vitamin B_{12} binder (transcobalamin I and III) increased

Clinical features
1. Incidence 1:100 000. Occurs predominantly in the middle-aged, with equal sex incidence
2. Onset—usually insidious

3. Common symptoms are due to:
   (i)   Anaemia—lethargy
   (ii) Splenomegaly (often massive)—dragging sensation, 'fullness', pain (often due to infarcts)
   (iii) Haemorrhage—from easy bruising to severe bleeding (usually late, when the platelet count is low)
4. Systemic symptoms—fever, sweats, and weight-loss with wasting may become features during course of disease
5. Other less common features include:
   (i)   Bone and joint pain
   (ii) Gout and/or urate renal stones
   (iii) Priapism, due to thrombosis of the corpus cavernosum
   (iv) Confusion/coma, due to cerebral leucostasis
6. Physical findings—splenomegaly, usually marked, is the most constant sign. Hepatomegaly is usually moderate

Treatment
1. Chemotherapy:
   (i)   Busulphan (alkylating agent)—the drug of choice in effecting controlled reduction in WBC and platelet counts, and reduction in spleen size. May cause prolonged marrow aplasia and permanent infertility
   (ii) Hydroxyurea (antimetabolite)—a useful alternative to busulphan, especially in younger patients worried about infertility
   (iii) Various agents alone or in combination have been tried in blast cell crisis with little success (see below)
2. α-interferon—the majority of patients show a reduction in leucocyte count in chronic phase with a reduction in the proportion of Ph positive metaphases (in some cases complete loss of Ph positivity)
3. Allogeneic bone marrow transplant—treatment of choice in first chronic phase for patients <55 years old with HLA-compatible donor. Results poor after blastic transformation
4. Radiotherapy—splenic irradiation, particularly for pain control
5. Splenectomy—of dubious value
6. Leucapheresis—beneficial in patients presenting with leucostasis, or in the treatment of CML in pregnancy (when cytotoxics contraindicated)

Course and prognosis
1. Median duration of chronic phase is $2\frac{1}{2}$–3 years
2. Progressive disease, with variable rapidity
   (i)   Blast cell crisis (similar to acute leukaemia)
   (ii) Slower transformation with proliferative variance—accelerated phase
3. Median survival is only slightly increased by conventional cytotoxic treatment (about 3 years); 50–75% cure rate with

ablative therapy and allogeneic BMT in first chronic phase (c.f. 15% in acute blastic transformation)

BLAST CELL TRANSFORMATION

Defined by the presence of > 30% blasts or blasts plus promyelocytes in bone marrow or peripheral blood:
1. Myeloid type (70%)—often unresponsive to chemotherapy; drugs as for AML may be given, though responses are usually short-lived
2. Lymphoid type (20–25%) associated with cALLA, TdT and Ia positivity. Some patients respond well to the agents typically active in ALL, e.g. vincristine and prednisolone
3. 5–10% have mixed myeloid and lymphoid markers

PH NEGATIVE CGL

Characteristic features include:
1. Occurrence in a younger age group
2. Less marked splenomegaly
3. Lower WBC, with no myelocyte, eosinophil or basophil proliferation
4. Monocytosis, with increased serum and urine lysozyme
5. Low platelet count (< 100 × 10^9/l) at presentation
6. More rapid evolution, less responsive to therapy

FURTHER ADVANCED READING

Berk P D et al 1986 Therapeutic recommendations in polycythaemia vera based on Polycythaemia Vera Study Group protocols. Seminars in Haematology 23, 132–143
Galton D A G (ed) 1977 The chronic leukaemias. Clinics in haematology 6, no 1. W B Saunders, London
Goldman J M (ed) 1987 Chronic myeloid leukaemia. Clinical haematology 1:4. Baillière Tindall, London

11. Secondary polycythaemia and thrombocythaemia

SECONDARY POLYCYTHAEMIA (ERYTHROCYTOSIS)

Definition
Absolute increase in red cell mass *not* due to a primary myeloproliferative process.

Pathogenesis
Either:
1. Stimulation of the humoral erythropoietic regulatory mechanism by hypoxia, i.e. 'compensatory'

or:

2. Inappropriate production of humoral factors which stimulate erythropoiesis

Haematology
1. Hb, RBC and PCV increased
2. Blood viscosity—increased
3. Bone marrow—erythroid hyperplasia. Iron stores may be depleted (especially in phlebotomised patients)

Other investigations
1. Arterial pO_2 reduced in hypoxic group
2. Red cell mass increased
3. Erythropoietin levels increased

Associations
1. Hypoxia ('appropriate' secretion of erythropoietin):
   (i) Residence at high altitude (viz: classic studies in the Andes)
   (ii) Chronic respiratory disease, e.g. severe obstructive airways disease
   (iii) Cardiac disease, especially congenital cyanotic, e.g. Eisenmenger's syndrome, Fallot's tetralogy
   (iv) Extreme obesity
   (v) Chronic carbon monoxide poisoning—e.g. in heavy tobacco

smokers (obstructive airways disease may be contributory factor)
(vi) High affinity haemoglobins
(vii) Congenital methaemoglobinaemia
2. Miscellaneous, mostly rare ('inappropriate' secretion of erythropoietin):
   (i) Renal disease, e.g. cystic disease, renal artery stenosis, carcinoma
   (ii) Cerebellar haemangioblastoma
   (iii) Various neoplasms, e.g. carcinoma of liver
   (iv) Uterine fibroids
   (v) Endocrine therapy with androgens

Diagnosis
Differentiation from polycythaemia rubra vera clinically is usually based on the particular features of these associated conditions and the absence of splenomegaly, leucocytosis and thrombocytosis; hypermetabolic symptoms are absent. Erythropoietin levels provide a valuable guide in investigation

Treatment
1. Of the underlying association/disease where possible
2. Venesection—when erythrocytosis and viscosity increases are marked. Careful assessment after a 'trial' of treatment is advisable; the aim is to maintain PCV < 0.5

APPARENT (RELATIVE) POLYCYTHAEMIA

Associations
These are various:
1. Dehydration (e.g. burns, enteritis), alcohol abuse and diuretic therapy
2. Hypertension, chronic stress (Gaisboeck's syndrome, polycythaemia of stress)

Laboratory findings
1. Raised Hb and PCV
2. Normal WBC and platelet count
3. Normal erythropoietin level
4. Normal red cell mass with reduced plasma volume, or upper normal range red cell mass with lower normal range plasma volume

Treatment
Of the associated disorder if identified, e.g. control hypertension, discontinue diuretics if possible. Venesection may have a role in some cases of relative polycythaemia associated with cardiovascular problems.

SECONDARY THROMBOCYTHAEMIA

To be distinguished from the primary myeloproliferative disorder.

Causes

1. Reactive to:
   (i)   Blood loss
   (ii) Haemolysis
2. Post-splenectomy
3. In association with:
   (i)   Malignant disease (carcinoma, lymphoma)
   (ii) Chronic inflammatory disease states, e.g. rheumatoid arthritis, ulcerative colititis, Crohn's disease
4. Following surgery or trauma
5. Infection
6. Exercise
7. Drugs, e.g. vincristine, steroids

12. Neutrophil abnormalities

NEUTROPENIA

Causes

1. Defective granulopoiesis
(i)   Ineffective, as in B_{12} and folate deficiencies, myelodysplasia
(ii) Secondary to a malignant proliferation (haematological or non-haematological)
(iii) Secondary to hypoplasia, e.g. drug-induced, aplastic anaemia

2. Removal from circulation
(i) Peripheral destruction, e.g. by immune mechanisms (disease- or drug-induced), hypersplenism
(ii) Shifts of neutrophils into the marginal pool. e.g. anaphylactic shock and toxaemias, neutropenia of Afro-Caribbeans (not 'true' neutropenias)

3. Miscellaneous and idiopathic
(i)   Infections:
      a. Bacterial—e.g. typhoid, paratyphoid, brucella
      b. Viral—e.g. viral hepatitis, infectious mononucleosis
      c. Protozoal—e.g. malaria
      d. Rickettsial—e.g. scrub typhus
(ii) Drug-induced:
      a. Predictable—dose-related, e.g. cyclophosphamide
      b. Immune e.g. amidopyrine
      c. Idiosyncratic e.g. chlorpromazine
(iii) Idiopathic—the majority are relatively benign, though cyclical neutropenia (often with recurrently low counts every 21–28 days) may be associated with periodic infections and mucosal ulceration. Occasional fatal neutropenias have been recorded

Clinical features
1. Susceptibility to infection—the risk depending on the degree and duration of neutropenia

2. Pyrexias and constitutional symptoms, with or without obvious infection
3. Infections ('opportunistic'):
   (i) Localised—e.g. oropharynx, skin, perianal region. Necrosis with ulceration common
   (ii) Generalised—septicaemias, e.g. due to Gram-negative bacteria. May be rapidly fatal
4. Features of associated disease

Treatment
1. Appropriate broad-spectrum antimicrobial agents— antibacterial, antifungal
2. Of the underlying cause

NEUTROPHIL FUNCTIONAL DEFECTS

Functional defects are probably more common than previously thought, but the significance of abnormal tests (the majority are carried out in vitro) is not always clear.

Basic physiology and biochemistry (see p.173)

CHRONIC GRANULOMATOUS DISEASE (CGD)

Genetics
X-linked recessive transmission (majority).

Pathology
1. The basic defect is failure of the metabolic burst following phagocytosis with little increase in oxygen consumption and inadequate hydrogen peroxide formation due to absence of cytochrome b_{245}
2. Defective intracellular killing of microorganisms (except bacteria which produce peroxide), e.g. staphylococci, *Aspergillus fumigatus*, *Candida albicans*

Haematology
1. No diagnostic abnormalities of indices or in film
2. CGD neutrophils fail to reduce nitroblue tetrazolium dye (NBT) (yellow) to formazan (blue-black) normally
3. Neutrophils show markedly decreased ability to kill bacteria and fungi in in vitro tests

Clinical features
1. Primarily affects males
2. Infections often occur early in childhood and may occur at any site
3. Granulomatous reactions are frequent later

4. Regional lymphadenopathy is common
5. Infections of particular importance:
   (i)   Pulmonary, often chronic
   (ii) Hepatic—abscesses, indolent infection
   (iii) In relation to the oropharynx and GI tract
   (iv) Osteomyelitis

Treatment
1. Appropriate antibiotic therapy for specific infections (the use of continuous antibiotics may encourage survival of resistant bacteria)
2. Transfusion of granulocytes from healthy donors in emergency situations
3. α-interferon

Prognosis
Improving with advances in treatment, but death in childhood likely.

CHEDIAK–HIGASHI SYNDROME

A rare disease with autosomal recessive transmission and the following features:
1. Granulocytes and precursors contain large inclusions due to coalescence of many primary granules. Neutropenia and thrombocytopenia are usually present
2. Chemotaxis, migration and intracellar killing of microorganisms defective. Function of lysosomal membrane appears abnormal; bacterial ingestion and lysosomal enzymes appear normal
3. Clinical associations include albinism, hepatosplenomegaly and lymphadenopathy
4. Usually fatal in early childhood from infection or haemorrhage; survivors have an increased risk of developing lymphomas

SCHWACHMAN'S SYNDROME

A rare disease with autosomal recessive transmission and the following features:
1. Chondrodysplasia with growth retardation, exocrine pancreatic dysfunction
2. Neutropenia and impaired neutrophil mobility

ENZYME DEFICIENCIES

Rarely of clinical significance as causes of impaired function, e.g. myeloperoxidase deficiency, severe glucose-6-phosphate dehydrogenase deficiency.

MORPHOLOGICAL VARIATIONS

PELGER-HÜET ANOMALY

1. Rare condition (autosomal dominant transmission)
2. Functionally normal bilobed neutrophils with 'pince-nez' nuclei. Homozygotes may have neutrophils with single round nuclei

Note: 'Pseudo-Pelger' cells are often seen in myelodysplasia, acute myeloid leukaemia and infectious mononucleosis, or can be drug-related, e.g. colchicine. Functional defects frequently associated.

MAY–HEGGLIN ANOMALY

1. Rare condition (autosomal dominant transmission)
2. Basophilic RNA inclusions (Döhle bodies) present in cytoplasm
3. Associated leucopenia, thrombocytopenia and giant platelets
4. Haemorrhagic problems may occur
5. Acquired form seen with infections, burns and pregnancy

ALDER-REILLY ANOMALY

1. Rare condition (autosomal recessive transmission)
2. Deep purple granules, due to an abnormality of polysaccharide storage, found in granulocytes, monocytes and lymphocytes
3. Neutrophils are functionally normal
4. Seen in association with gargoylism (Hurler's syndrome) and amaurotic familiar idiocy (Tay–Sachs disease)

MISCELLANEOUS

Defects of chemotaxis, phagocytosis and killing of microorganisms may occur in a wide variety of disease states, but particularly haematological malignancies. The clinical significance is not always clear.

FURTHER ADVANCED READING

Klebanoff S J, Clark R A 1978 The neutrophil: function and clinical disorders. North Holland Publishing Company, Oxford

13. Leucocytosis and leuco-erythroblastosis

Definition

An increase in numbers of circulating leucocytes to greater than $11 \times 10^9/l$.

NEUTROPHILIA ($> 7.5 \times 10^9/l$)

Commonest cause of leucocytosis.

Often associated with toxic granulation, 'shift to the left' with band forms and occasional metamyelocytes, and Döhle bodies. Seen in association with the following conditions:

1. Acute infection—e.g. abscesses, septicaemia
2. Tissue damage—e.g. myocardial infarction, burns, gangrene, vasculitis
3. Neoplasia
4. Haemorrhage and haemolysis
5. Chronic myeloid leukaemia, chronic myelomonocytic leukaemia, myelofibrosis
6. Metabolic disorders—e.g. diabetes, gout, uraemia
7. Drugs—e.g. prednisolone, lithium
8. Strenuous exercise

EOSINOPHILIA ($> 0.44 \times 10^9/l$)

Seen in association with:

1. Allergy—e.g. hay fever, asthma, urticaria
2. Parasitic infestations, especially if there is tissue invasion
3. Skin disease—e.g. eczema, dermatitis herpetiformis, psoriasis
4. Myeloproliferative diseases, e.g. PRV, CML, chronic eosinophilic leukaemia
5. Neoplasia—especially Hodgkin's disease (5% patients)
6. Miscellaneous—e.g. polyarteritis nodosa, pulmonary eosinophilia (± parasitic infiltration; Loeffler's syndrome), sarcoidosis, hypereosinophilic syndrome, post-irradiation

MONOCYTOSIS ($> 0.8 \times 10^9$/l)

Seen in association with the following conditions:
1. Infection—e.g. tuberculosis, brucellosis, subacute bacterial endocarditis, typhus, malaria, kala-azar
2. Inflammatory disorders—e.g. rheumatoid arthritis, SLE, Crohn's disease, ulcerative colitis
3. Neoplasia
4. Haematological malignancy—e.g. CMML, AML—M_4 and M_6

BASOPHILIA ($> 0.1 \times 10^9$/l)

Seen in association with:
1. Myxoedema
2. Chickenpox
3. Myeloproliferative disorders, especially PRV or CML (may herald blastic transformation)

LYMPHOCYTOSIS ($> 3.5 \times 10^9$/l)

Seen in association with:
1. Acute infections—e.g. infectious mononucleosis, rubella, pertussis, mumps, infectious lymphocytosis
2. Chronic infections—e.g. brucellosis, tuberculosis, syphilis, hepatitis
3. Haematological disorders—e.g. chronic lymphatic leukaemia, hairy cell leukaemia, chronic T-cell lymphocytosis (large granular lymphocytes)

LEUKAEMOID REACTIONS

Extremely high leucocyte counts ($> 50 \times 10^9$/l) seen in non-leukaemic conditions, simulating myeloid or lymphatic leukaemia. Seen in association with severe infections, especially in children and splenectomised patients. Differentiation from chronic myeloid leukaemia is important (see Table 13.1).

Table 13.1

	Leukaemoid reaction	Chronic myeloid leukaemia
Toxic granulation	Prominent	Absent
LAP score	Very high	Very low
Cytogenetic analysis	Normal	Ph chromosome (usual)
Clinical findings	Signs of infection	Splenomegaly

LEUCO-ERYTHROBLASTIC REACTIONS

LEUCO-ERYTHROBLASTIC ANAEMIA

Definition

An abnormal peripheral blood picture characterised by the presence of immature myeloid and erythroid cells, due to replacement of normal haematopoietic tissue in bone marrow by abnormal cells/tissue.

Mechanisms

Not simply a 'space-occupying' phenomenon—there is poor correlation between haematological changes and the degree of marrow abnormality.

Causes

1. Metastatic cancer, e.g. lung, breast, prostate, kidney, thyroid
2. Myelofibrosis (see p.92)
3. Myelomatosis (see p.80)
4. Malignant lymphomas (see p.59)
5. Gaucher's disease, Niemann–Pick disease
6. Megaloblastic anaemia (see p.9)
7. Granulomatous infections, e.g. tuberculosis
8. Osteopetrosis

All these conditions may be associated with *other* haematological changes and the following features refer to 'typical' leuco-erythroblastic anaemia.

Haematology

1. Anaemia, usually mild-moderate normochromic, normocytic
2. WBC—usually normal or increased
3. Blood film:
   (i) Red cells show anisocytosis and poikilocytosis (especially in some metastatic cancers). Nucleated red cells are present, often numerous
   (ii) White cells show a left shift with metamyelocytes, myelocytes and even myeloblasts present
4. ESR—often increased
5. Bone marrow—aspirate may be normal or contain characteristic cells (or microorganisms, in tuberculosis). A trephine biopsy is more likely to be diagnostic

Radiology

May be of diagnostic value, e.g. characteristic bone lesions of myelomatosis/carcinomatosis.

The cause may not be obvious and detailed investigation is then required.

Clinical significance
In cancer, indicates disseminated disease, often making surgical excision of the primary unjustifiable.

GAUCHER'S DISEASE

Genetics
Autosomal recessive transmission. Rare.

Pathology
1. β-glucosidase deficiency leads to accumulation of glucocerebroside
2. Gaucher cells (in spleen, liver, marrow)—atypical histiocytes with a fibrillar 'onion-skin' appearance due to glucocerebroside content

Haematology
Features of hypersplenism and/or leuco-erythroblastic anaemia with Gaucher cells in marrow (and sometimes in blood film).

Treatment
Splenectomy/BMT may be indicated

Clinical features
Cutaneous pigmentation, hepatosplenomegaly (often massive), neuropathies and skeletal defects. A variable course, but survival into adult life is usual.

NIEMANN–PICK DISEASE

Genetics
Autosomal recessive transmission. Rare.

Pathology
1. Sphingomyelinase deficiency with accumulation of sphingomyelin
2. Characteristic cells (in spleen, liver, marrow, CNS) have 'foamy' vacuolated cytoplasms ± 'sea-blue' histiocytes

Haematology
Hypersplenism less common than in Gaucher's disease. Characteristic cells in blood film and marrow.

Clinical features
Hepatosplenomegaly and CNS involvement. Usually fatal in infancy, but early BMT may prolong survival.

14. Acute leukaemia

Definition
A malignant neoplasm characterised by disorderly, clonal proliferation of immature haemopoietic cells with acute onset.

Aetiological factors

1. Genetics
(i)   There is a slight familial tendency overall (*Note*: high concordance in monozygotic twins)
(ii) Chromosome abnormalities (quantitative/qualitative) in about 50% of patients. A high incidence, 20–30 × expected, in mongolism (trisomy of chromosome 21)

2. Ionising radiation
(i)   Excessive exposure in therapy of, e.g., ankylosing spondylitis, malignant disease
(ii) Nuclear explosions/accidents, as at Hiroshima, Chernobyl

3. Drugs
Prolonged chemotherapy, e.g. with alkylating agents, *especially* if combined with radiotherapy, in the treatment of malignant diseases.

4. Immune status
The incidence of leukaemia is increased in immunosuppressed individuals.

5. Viruses
Retroviruses, implicated in some lymphoproliferative disorders— e.g. HTLV I causes adult T-cell leukaemia/lymphoma (ATLL), HTLV II is associated with hairy cell leukaemia—but viral associations in the acute leukaemias not established.

Classification
Broadly into acute lymphoblastic leukaemia (ALL) or acute

myeloblastic leukaemia (AML or ANLL). Important prognostically, and for treatment which differs for each type. Subcategories are defined by analysis of morphology, cytochemistry, cell markers and cytogenetics (see Tables 14.1–4)

Table 14.1   Morphology—FAB (French–American–British) classification

ALL	AML
L_1— Small, monomorphic, high N/C* ratio, indistinct nucleoli	M_0—Undifferentiated
	M_1—Myeloblastic without maturation
L_2— Large, heterogeneous, lower N/C ratio, prominent nucleoli	
	M_2—Myeloblastic with maturation
L_3— Large, low N/C ratio, basophilic vacuolated cytoplasm (Burkitt cells)	M_3—Hypergranular promyelocytic
	—Hypogranular variant
	M_4—Myelomonocytic
	—M_4Eo with marrow eosinophilia
	M_5—Monoblastic (M_{5a})
	—Promonocytic/monocytic (M_{5b})
	M_6—Erythroleukaemia
	M_7—Megakaryoblastic

*N/C = Nuclear/cytoplasmic

Table 14.2   Cytochemistry

ALL		AML	
Peroxidase	—Negative	Peroxidase	—Positive, M_1–M_5 (some)
Sudan Black	—Negative	Sudan Black	—Positive, M_1–M_5 (some)
PAS	—Block positivity, cALL	PAS	—Diffuse/granular positivity, M_2–M_7
Esterase	—Negative	Esterase	—Non-specific-positive, monocytes
Acid phosphatase	—Localised positivity, T-ALL		—Specific-positive, granulocytes
		Acid phosphatase	—Diffuse positivity, M_2–M_6

Table 14.3 Cell markers and cluster differentiation (immunophenotypes)

	ALL						AML					
	Null	cALL	preB	B-ALL	T-ALL		M_0	M_1	$M_{2/3}$	$M_{4/5}$	M_6	M_7
TdT	+	+	+	−	+	TdT	−/+	−/+	−	−	−	−
CD_3	−	−	−	−	+	CD_7	−	−	−	−	−	−
CD_7	−	−	−	−	+	CD_{13}	+	+	+	+	+	+
CD_{10}	−	+	+	−/+	−	CD_{14}	−	−	−	+	−	−
$CD_{13/33}$	−	−	−	−	−	CD_{19}	−	−	−	−	−	−
CD_{19}	+	+	+	+	−	CD_{33}	−/+	+	+	+	−/+	+
CD_{22}	+	+	+	+	−	CD_{42}	−	−	−	−	−	+
Cytμ	−	−	+	+/−	−	CD_{44}	−	−	−	−	+	−

Table 14.4 Cytogenetics

ALL	AML
t(9,22) — assoc. with 2–20% cases of c-ALL	t(15,17) — M_3 and variant
t(4,11) — High WBC — L_2 morphology	t(8,21)—M_2 and M_4
t(8,14) — assoc. with B-ALL — L_3 morphology	inv 16—M_4Eo
	5q-, 7q- Trisomy 8

ACUTE LYMPHOBLASTIC LEUKAEMIA (ALL)

Pathogenesis
1. Malignant transformation of a clone of precursor cells
2. Proliferation of lymphoblasts in bone marrow
3. Interference with normal haemopoiesis
4. Variable appearance of blast cells in peripheral blood
5. Widespread invasion of various tissues and organs by blast cells:
   (i)   Lymph nodes and spleen
   (ii) Liver
   (iii) Central nervous system
   (iv) Testis and ovary

Haematology
1. Anaemia usually normocytic, normochromic

2. WBC—usually increased, with many blast cells, though counts often < 10 × 10^9/l in children (higher in T-cell ALL). Variable neutropenia
3. Blood film:
   (i) Lymphoblasts, with characteristic features (see Table 14.1):
       a. Nuclear/cytoplasmic ratio high
       b. Cytoplasm usually agranular
       c. Nucleus may be cleft but not indented or twisted
       d. Nucleoli—often one or two
       e. Peroxidase and Sudan Black negative
       f. PAS positive—coarse granules, typically
       g. TdT (enzyme, terminal deoxynucleotidyl transferase)— increased/positive (majority of patients but not B-ALL)
   (ii) Other cell lines—morphology often normal
4. Thrombocytopenia usual and may be marked (platelets <50 × 10^9/l)
5. Bone marrow—hyperplastic, normal cells being replaced by proliferating blast cells
6. CSF—blasts may be present (demonstrated by 'cytospin')
7. Acquired clotting abnormalities, e.g. DIC (rarely severe)

Biochemistry
1. Plasma urate levels often increased—reflecting the proliferating leukaemic cell mass
2. Increased CSF protein in CNS involvement

Radiology
1. Chest—changes often due to infection, much less commonly to leukaemic infiltration. Mediastinal mass often demonstrable in T-ALL
2. Skeleton—lesions, usually osteolytic, are common in children, much less so in adults

Clinical features
1. Predominantly (90%) children under 14 years of age. Slight male preponderance
2. Commonly presents with symptoms of anaemia, e.g. tiredness and malaise, often compounded by symptoms of infection
3. Sequelae of neutropenia:
   (i) Fever
   (ii) Overt infections, frequently oral initially
4. Sequelae of thrombocytopenia:
   (i) Petechiae
   (ii) Purpura
   (iii) Epistaxis and bleeding gums
   (iv) Gastrointestinal haemorrhage
   (v) Cerebral haemorrhage

5. Bone pain, especially in children
6. Lymph node enlargement—more pronounced in children than adults and particularly in T-ALL, when it may cause SVC obstruction
7. Hepatomegaly and splenomegaly—usually slight (more prominent in T-ALL)
8. Symptoms and signs secondary to CNS infiltration:
   (i) Headaches, vomiting, visual changes and papilloedema (due to raised intracranial pressure)
   (ii) Cranial nerve palsies

Treatment
1. Remission induction. Aim is to achieve complete remission (CR), i.e. <5% blasts in normocellular marrow:
   (i) Vincristine and prednisolone commonly induce remission within 4–6 weeks in 90% of prepubertal patients
   (ii) Additional active agents are given to enhance overall response rates. The more intensive regimens, which include daunorubicin, L-asparaginase, methotrexate and cyclophosphamide, are indicated in poor risk childhood ALL, B-ALL and adults. Associated with higher early morbidity and mortality, but remission rates of 95–98%
2. Consolidation:
   (i) Various early and/or late intensification schedules (including vincristine, prednisolone, daunorubicin, etoposide, cytosine arabinoside and 6-thioguanine)—currently being evaluated
   (ii) CNS prophylaxis—reduces risk of CNS relapse from 50% to 5%
      a. Intrathecal methotrexate—6 doses (standard)
      b. Cranial irradiation (18–24 Gy). Causes transient somnolence and lethargy after 6 weeks. Should be avoided if bone marrow transplantation is planned (intrathecal methotrexate regimen may be intensified to compensate)
3. Maintenance—with monthly pulses of vincristine and prednisolone, weekly methotrexate and daily 6-mercaptopurine for 18–24 months
4. Supportive—(see p.115)
5. Bone marrow transplantation (see p.122)

Prognosis
1. Best prognosis is in children aged 2–9 (50–75% cure); cf. adults (35% cure with chemotherapy; 45–50% with allogeneic BMT)
2. Of poor prognosis:
   (i) High pre-treatment WBC ($>50 \times 10^9/l$) and extensive extramedullary infiltration (especially CNS)

(ii)   Significant lymphadenopathy/hepatosplenomegaly
(iii) Slow cytoreduction during induction
(iv)   B-ALL (carries particularly bad prognosis)

ACUTE MYELOBLASTIC AND MYELOMONOCYTIC LEUKAEMIAS (AML AND AMML)

Pathogenesis
Essentially as for acute lymphoblastic leukaemia, except that:
1. Infiltration of lymphoid tissue is generally less common
2. Infiltration of the typical 'refuge' sites—CNS and testis—is unusual
3. Infiltration of gums, oral mucous membranes and skin is frequent in myelomonocytic leukaemia

Haematology
1. Anaemia usually normochromic, normocytic
2. WBC—less than 4×10^9/l in approx. 50%, normal in 20% and increased in 30% of patients (usually due to circulating blast cells)
3. Thrombocytopenia common and may be marked (platelets $<50 \times 10^9$/l)
4. Blood film (see Table 14.1):
   (i)   Myeloblasts, with characteristic features:
         a. Nuclear/cytoplasmic ratio not high
         b. Cytoplasmic granules often apparent (large aggregates form Auer rods)
         c. Nuclei—indented and twisted in the myelomonocytic form
         d. Nucleoli—often 3–5
         e. Frequently but not invariably peroxidase and Sudan Black positive
         f. PAS—diffuse/granular positivity
         g. Characteristic esterase pattern
         h. TdT low/negative
   (ii) Red cells—anisocytosis and poikilocytosis, occasional circulating erythroblasts
   (iii) Neutrophils variably show some dysplastic features, e.g. hypogranularity and the acquired Pelger–Hüet anomaly
   (iv) Monocytes and promonocytes (sometimes atypical) often comprise >20% of nucleated cells in AMML
5. Bone marrow—usually hyperplastic due to proliferating myeloblasts (with monocytic component in AMML)
6. Acquired clotting abnormalities, e.g. secondary to hepatic infiltration or DIC

Biochemistry
1. Plasma urate levels often increased

2. Serum lysozyme (muramidase) increased in myelomonocytic form
3. Hypokalaemia—M_4, M_6.

Clinical features
1. Occurs at all ages, but predominantly in adults
2. Symptoms of anaemia ⎫
3. Sequelae of neutropenia ⎬ as for ALL
4. Sequelae of thrombocytopenia ⎭
5. Lymphadenopathy—slight or absent
6. Hepatomegaly and splenomegaly—slight or absent
7. Gum hypertrophy especially in the myelomonocytic form
8. CNS involvement much less likely than in ALL; more likely to be associated with M_4 EO variant or M_5

Treatment
1. Remission induction—70–80+% patients achieve remission with combinations of daunorubicin, cytosine arabinoside and 6-thioguanine (DAT) or etoposide (ADE). Drugs are less selective than in ALL regimes, causing profound pancytopenia
2. Consolidation—with the same/alternative induction regimens and combinations of m-AMSA, cytosine arabinoside, etoposide and mitozantrone
3. Maintenance—of limited proven benefit, increasingly omitted. Role of α-interferon being evaluated
4. Bone marrow transplantation:
   (i) Allogeneic ⎫
   (ii) Autologous in first/second CR ⎬ see p.122
5. Elderly patients with AML—less intensive approaches are the subject of therapeutic studies. Results awaited

Prognosis
1. 20–25% 5-year survival with standard chemotherapy; cf. 50% with allogeneic BMT
2. Poor prognostic features include:
   (i)   Poor performance status ± old age
   (ii) High WBC/thrombocytopenia ($< 25 \times 10^9$/l) at presentation
   (iii) Certain chromosomal abnormalities (see Table 14.1)
   (iv) Underlying myelodysplasia
   (v)   Secondary leukaemia, e.g. following previous chemo-radiotherapy

Supportive therapy
1. Basic considerations
(i) Depression of normal haemopoiesis is a consequence of chemotherapy and inevitable in the successful induction

therapy of AML. Generally less severe in the treatment of ALL
(ii) Immunosuppression due to the disease is compounded by the effects of chemotherapy on cellular immunity
(iii) The disruptive effects of drugs on mucosae (notably of mouth and gut) can easily lead to bacteraemia and septicaemia
(iv) Patients may die rapidly of:
    a. Overwhelming infection
    b. Catastrophic haemorrhage (e.g. cerebral)
(v) Opportunistic infective microorganisms include:
    a. *Staphylococcus aureus* (relatively easily treated) and coagulase negative staphylococci (often in relation to central venous lines)
    b. Gram-negative bacteria, e.g. *E. coli, Klebsiella pneumoniae* and *Pseudomonas aeruginosa*—resistant organisms can prove a problem
    c. Fungi—*Candida* spp. *Aspergillus* spp.
    d. Protozoa—*Pneumocystis carinii*
    e. Viruses—e.g. measles, varicella zoster cause 5% mortality in remission in childhood ALL. Prophylactic specific hyperimmune globulin should be given after exposure

2. Prophylaxis
(i) Skin and mouth hygiene (e.g. antiseptic mouthwashes)
(ii) Continuous oral antifungal agent (e.g. nystatin)
(iii) Reduction in gut flora (partial gut sterilisation is possible using oral antibiotics)
(iv) Continuous specific antibiotic cover—co-trimoxazole in ALL reduces the incidence of pneumocystis
(v) Daily platelet transfusions in patients with very low counts

3. Empiric
Early treatment of the pyrexial neutropenic patient (before any organism is isolated) may be life-saving. A valuable combination with broad cover is piperacillin plus an aminoglycoside (e.g. gentamicin).

4. Specific and non-specific
(i) Appropriate antimicrobial therapy should be given for the particular opportunistic infection
(ii) Blood products, as indicated. Granulocyte transfusions may be of value (see p.159)

OTHER ACUTE MYELOID LEUKAEMIA VARIANTS

These deserve brief consideration in order to illustrate the spectrum of disease.

ACUTE UNDIFFERENTIATED LEUKAEMIA (Mo)

1. Morphologically resemble L_2 blasts
2. Cytochemistry negative by standard methods; peroxidase activity at ultrastructural level
3. Markers: TdT may be positive; other lymphoid markers negative. $CD_{13/33}$ (myeloid) markers positive
4. Clinical features and treatment—as for AML/AMML
5. Course and prognosis as for AML/AMML

ACUTE HYPERGRANULAR PROMYELOCYTIC LEUKAEMIA (M_3)

1. Proliferation of abnormal hypergranulated promyelocytes
2. Haematology:
   (i) Promyelocytes contain abundant, abnormal cytoplasmic granules and bundles of Auer rods ('faggots')
   (ii) May present with low WBC and pancytopenia
   (iii) Coagulation abnormalities (notably DIC) occur and may be severe during induction treatment
3. Clinical features—increased haemorrhagic tendency, otherwise as for AML
4. Treatment:
   (i) Haemorrhagic problems may require treatment with heparin, platelets, other blood products and antifibrinolytics
   (ii) Chemotherapy as for AML
5. Course and prognosis—relatively good prognosis if CR achieved without fatal haemorrhagic problems.

ACUTE HYPOGRANULAR PROMYELOCYTIC LEUKAEMIA (M_3 VARIANT)

1. Promyelocytes have bilobed or reniform nuclei and occasional granules, and resemble M_6
2. Usually presents with very high WBC (up to $200 \times 10^9/l$); haemorrhagic problems as in M_3
3. Treatment, course and prognosis—as in M_3

ACUTE MONOCYTIC LEUKAEMIA (M_5)

1. Proliferation predominantly or, entirely, of the monocytic series
2. Haematology—essentially as for AMML but with differences in cytochemistry, particularly the esterase characteristics (see Table 14.1)
3. Serum lysozyme (muramidase) usually greatly increased; may cause renal tubular dysfunction and hypokalaemia
4. Clinical features—essentially as for AMML, often with very

pronounced gingival hypertrophy. CNS infiltration more likely than in AML/AMML
5. Treatment as for AML/AMML (though prognosis worse)

ERYTHROLEUKAEMIA (di Guglielmo's syndrome) (M_6)

1. Proliferation involving both erythroid and granulocytic series—$> 50\%$ erythroblasts and $> 30\%$ non-erythroid cells are myeloblastic
2. Haematology—erythroblasts show dysplastic features, usually PAS positivity and often sideroblastic change
3. Clinical features and treatment—essentially as for AML/AMML (though prognosis worse)

ACUTE MEGAKARYOBLASTIC LEUKAEMIA (M_7)

1. Proliferation of megakaryoblasts which may resemble lymphoblasts ± cytoplasmic budding; platelet peroxidase activity demonstrable by electron microscopy
2. Haematology—may present with low WBC and marrow fibrosis
3. Clinical features and treatment—essentially as for AML/AMML (though prognosis worse)

MYELODYSPLASTIC SYNDROMES (MDS)

Primary—arising 'de novo'
Secondary—arising after treatment with chemotherapy ± radiotherapy

Primary MDS
A range of acquired clonal disorders characterised by:
1. Ineffective haemopoiesis with peripheral cytopenias despite a hypercellular marrow
2. Morphologically and functionally abnormal haemopoietic precursors
   (i) Erythroid:
       a. Nuclear irregularity/multinuclearity
       b. Intercellular bridges—nuclear/cytoplasmic
       c. Defective haemoglobinisation
       d. Macrocytosis (despite normal B_{12} and folate levels)
       e. Ring sideroblasts ±
   (ii) Myeloid:
       a. Hypogranular or agranular neutrophils
       b. Bilobed nuclei—acquired Pelger–Hüet anomaly
       c. Irregular granularity of myeloid precursors
       d. Blasts (±)

(iii) Megakaryocytic: mononuclear micromegakaryocytes; megakaryocyte fragments may be seen in peripheral blood
3. Chromosomal abnormalities common e.g. 5q–, 7q–, Trisomy 8
4. Potential for leukaemic transformation, usually into AML

Classification (FAB) (see Table 14.5)
1. Refractory anaemia (RA)
2. Refractory anaemia with sideroblasts (RAS)
3. Refractory anaemia with excess blasts (RAEB)
4. Refractory anaemia with excess blasts in transformation (RAEB-t)
5. Chronic myelomonocytic leukaemia (CMML)

Haematology
1. Cytopenias, often pancytopenia
2. Blood film—dysplastic features, e.g. abnormal red cells, hypogranular neutrophils, Pelger–Hüet forms; increased monocytes in CMML
3. Bone marrow—features of particular type of MDS with increasing blast cells in leukaemic transformation

Clinical features
1. Typically occur in middle and old age
2. Sequelae of the cytopenias—anaemia, infection, haemorrhage
3. Haemosiderosis, a consequence of multiple blood transfusions

Treatment
Chiefly supportive:
1. Blood and platelet transfusions
2. Prompt treatment of infections
3. Tranexamic acid may ameliorate haemorrhagic tendency
4. No specific chemotherapy—agents which promote cell differentiation in vitro disappointing in vivo as yet; low-dose cytosine arabinoside may produce haematological responses; cis-retinoic acid and vitamin D also being evaluated
5. Chemotherapy as for AML/AMML may be given for frank leukaemic transformation—responses with reversion to pre-existing dysplastic state may be achieved but often transient
6. Bone marrow transplantation—allogeneic BMT in younger patients offers the best prospect of prolonged survival
7. Chelation of iron with desferrioxamine—programmes for long-term treatment may be indicated in patients requiring frequent blood transfusions

Table 14.5 Classification of MDS

	RA	RAS	RAEB	RAEBt	CMML
% Blasts in blood	<1	<1	<5	>5	<1
% Blasts in marrow	<5	<5	5–20	21–29	5–20
Monocyte count (×10^9/l) in blood	<1	<1	<1	<1	>1
Ring sideroblasts (% of nucleated cells)	<15	>15	<15	<15	<15
Leukaemic transformation (%)	15	10	40	60	30
Median survival (months)	30	75	10	5	10
Treatment	Supportive (i) Transfusion ± desferrioxamine (ii) antibiotics (iii) platelets	Supportive ± pyridoxine	Supportive ± differentiating agents	Supportive chemotherapy allogeneic BMT	Supportive ± chemotherapy

chemotherapy ⎱ in young patients

Course and prognosis
Depends on the type of MDS but, in general terms:
1. Morbidity and deaths largely attributable to the refractory cytopenias:
   (i) Directly, e.g. haemorrhage
   (ii) Indirectly, e.g. transfusion-related haemosiderosis
2. Overall leukaemic transformation and related death occur in a minority of patients

FURTHER ADVANCED READING

Catovsky D (ed) 1991 The leukaemic cell 2nd edn. Churchill Livingstone, Edinburgh

Schmalzl F, Mufti G J (eds) 1991 Myelodysplastic syndromes. Springer Verlag, New York

Scott C S (ed) 1989 Leukaemia cytochemistry. Principles and practice. Ellis Horwood Ltd, Chichester

Whittaker J A, Delamore I W (eds) 1989 Leukaemia. Blackwell Scientific Publications, Oxford

15. Bone marrow transplantation (BMT)

Rationale
1. Standard chemotherapy regimens are limited to sublethal doses to allow marrow regeneration between courses
2. BMT allows ablative chemotherapy ± radiotherapy (with elimination of leukaemic clone) followed by 'rescue' with healthy donor stem cells (3×10^8/kg recipient)

Types
1. Allogeneic—HLA identical donor either sibling or matched unrelated donor (MUD)
2. Syngeneic—identical twin donor
3. Autologous—rescue with patient's own remission marrow harvested and stored prior to ablative therapy

Indications (allogeneic BMT)
In patients ≤55 years with HLA-identical donor:
1. AML—in 1st CR
2. ALL—poor risk in 1st CR
        good risk in 2nd CR
3. Severe aplastic anaemia
4. CGL in 1st chronic phase
5. MDS
6. Thalassaemia major (children)
7. Others—e.g. Fanconi's syndrome, storage disorders (children)

Complications
1. *Directly related to chemotherapy ± radiotherapy*
(i) Early (days):
   a. Nausea and vomiting
   b. Mucositis—sore mouth, diarrhoea, abdominal pain
   c. Haemorrhagic cystitis—preventable by routine administration of 2-mercaptoethane sulphonate (MESNA) with cyclophosphamide
(ii) Intermediate (weeks):
   a. Radiation somnolence (transient)

b. Organ damage—lungs (fibrosis), kidneys, liver, heart
c. Alopecia—may be permanent after busulphan

(iii) Late (months/years):
   a. Infertility—sperm cryopreservation should be considered and offered if appropriate before starting any chemotherapy prior to BMT
   b. Endocrine problems
      — hypothyroidism
      — early menopause
      — osteoporosis
      (Treat with replacement therapy as required)
   c. Cataracts (amenable to later surgery)

2. Myelosuppression (for 4–6 weeks post-BMT)

(i)   Anaemia ⎤ Blood and platelets should be irradiated
(ii) Thrombocytopenia ⎦ to prevent GvHD (see below)
(iii) Infections
   a. Bacterial—risk reduced by reversed barrier nursing, gut sterilisation
   b. Viral—especially CMV, herpes simplex, herpes zoster and measles; measures to reduce risk include use of CMV-negative blood products, acyclovir
   c. Protozoal—*Pneumocystis* pneumonia; preventable with cotrimoxazole prophylaxis

3. Graft-versus-host disease (GvHD)

(i)   Immunocompetent donor T lymphocytes recognise recipient antigens as foreign. Not seen in syngeneic or autologous BMT. May be fatal
(ii) Acute GvHD (<6 weeks post-BMT):
   a. Fever
   b. Skin—itchy, red, maculopapular rash on palms, soles and trunk. May become generalised with blisters, erythroderma and desquamation
   c. Liver—hepatitis
   d. Gut—profuse watery, green 'mint-sauce' diarrhoea ± haemorrhage
   e. Lung—increases risk of viral pneumonitis
(iii) Chronic GvHD (>6 weeks post-BMT):
   a. Skin pigmentation, contractures, scleroderma, lichen planus
   b. Gut—chronic diarrhoea, malabsorption
(iv) 'Graft v leukaemia' (GvL) effect:
   a. Donor T lymphocytes exert a cytotoxic effect against residual recipient leukaemia cells
   b. Better cure rate in patients who survive having had GvHD
(v)   GvHD prevention:
   a. Immunosuppressive therapy with cyclosporin/methotrexate after allogeneic BMT

  b. T-cell depletion of donor marrow with monoclonal
     antibodies. Reduces GvHD risk, but associated with
     increased risk of graft failure and leukaemic relapse
     (*especially* CGL)
(vi) GvHD treatment:
   a. Supportive—i.v. fluids, blood products
   b. Steroids—i.v. methylprednisolone e.g. 1.5 g daily × 3 ± oral
      prednisolone thereafter
   c. Azathioprine
   d. Thalidomide—effective in suppressing chronic GvHD

Prognosis (leukaemias)

Allogeneic BMT	— 40–50% probable cure rates
Syngeneic/autologous	— 30–40% probable cure rates
cf. Standard chemotherapy	— 20–25% 5-year survival (very few cures)

FURTHER ADVANCED READING

Champlin R E, Gale R P (eds) 1990 New strategies in bone marrow
   transplantation. Wiley-Liss, New York
Prentice H G, Brenner M K 1988 Recent advances in bone marrow
   transplantation in the treatment of leukaemia. In: Hoffbrand A V (ed)
   Recent advances in haematology 5. Churchill Livingstone, Edinburgh

16. Haemorrhagic diseases

Definition
Haemostatic defects resulting in pathological haemorrhage from intact blood vessels or excessive haemorrhage from ruptured blood vessels.

Basic physiology
Normal haemostasis comprises four principal components:
1. Vascular:
    (i)   Vasoconstriction
    (ii) Release of thromboplastin and prostacylin
2. Platelet:
    (i)   Adherence to subendothelial connective tissue
    (ii) Release of ADP and prostaglandin intermediates
    (iii) Aggregation of platelets to form a primary haemostatic plug
3. Fibrin:
    (i)   Production by activation of intrinsic/extrinsic clotting systems
    (ii) Deposition stabilises platelet plug—fibrin clot formation
4. Fibrinolytic:
    Limitation of the extent of clot formation—a 'protective' mechanism

Basic pathologies
1. Vascular abnormalities
2. Quantitative/qualitative platelet deficiencies
3. Defective coagulation mechanisms
4. Increased fibrinolysis

VASCULAR DEFECTS

Basic features
1. Can be inherited or acquired
2. Underlying lesions are of two main types:
    (i) Abnormal perivascular connective tissue—inadequate vessel support
    (ii) Intrinsically abnormal or damaged vessel wall

3. Spontaneous or post-traumatic bleeding, primarily into skin
4. Anaemia is infrequent, usually mild but occasionally severe, e.g. in hereditary haemorrhagic telangiectasia
5. WBC and platelets are usually normal
6. Standard screening clotting tests and bleeding time are normal

HEREDITARY HAEMORRHAGIC TELANGIECTASIA (Osler–Rendu–Weber syndrome)

Genetics
Autosomal dominant transmission.

Pathology
Multiple dilatations of small vessels (telangiectasia) in skin and mucous membranes (e.g. in nose and mouth) but *also* at other sites, e.g. liver, brain, lungs.

Clinical features
1. Symptoms, e.g. epistaxes, usually occur relatively late, i.e. during 2nd–3rd decade. The severity varies considerably between patients, but tends to increase with age
2. Typical lesions blanch on pressure, increase in size with age and bleed spontaneously or following trauma

Complication
Chronic blood loss may result in iron deficiency anaemia.

Treatment
Iron therapy/transfusions may be indicated. Cautery may reduce epistaxes

EHLERS–DANLOS SYNDROME

Genetics
Autosomal dominant transmission.

Pathology
Collagen defect (quantitative/qualitative), resulting in defective, fragile vessels and supportive tissue.

Clinical features
1. Typically, hyperelastic skin and hyperextensible joints
2. Mild haemorrhagic tendency. Subcutaneous haematomas occur and these may calcify

SCURVY

Aetiology
Vitamin C deficiency secondary to dietary inadequacies (e.g. in the old and neglected or with overcooking of food).

Pathology
Vascular fragility due to defective intercellular 'cement' secondary to failure of hydroxylation of collagen and elastin.

Clinical features
1. Bleeds—into skin (petechiae, purpura) and e.g. muscle
2. Hyperkeratotic hair follicles, with 'corkscrew' hairs
3. Swollen gums, especially interdental papillae—'scurvy buds'
4. Bone tenderness (children) due to subperiostial haemorrhage
5. Hess test may be positive

Biochemistry
White cell ascorbate is reduced.

Treatment
Vitamin C produces prompt resolution.

HENOCH–SCHÖNLEIN PURPURA

Aetiology
Presumed hypersensitivity reaction to e.g. streptococcal or viral infection, drugs or foodstuffs (particularly seafood).

Pathology
Widespread 'inflammation' of small vessels with perivascular cellular reaction, increased vascular permeability and exudation/haemorrhage; due to immune complex deposition with subsequent complement activation.

Clinical features
1. Commonest in childhood and adolescence
2. Purpuric lesions, often large and confluent, typically on buttocks and extensor surfaces of arms and legs
3. Colicky abdominal pain (due to extravasation from small vessels in gut wall). Rarely, intussusception
4. Joint pains ± periarticular swelling
5. Haematuria and proteinuria ± oedema

Treatment
No specific therapy. Corticosteroids and dapsone may give symptomatic relief.

Course and prognosis
Usually benign and self-limiting. Chronic renal insufficiency
develops in a minority (2–3%).

SIMPLE EASY BRUISING

Basic features
1. No apparent cause
2. Seen predominantly in otherwise healthy females
3. Bruises—chiefly on the legs
4. No effective treatment

SENILE PURPURA

Basic features
1. Due to atrophy of subcutaneous vascular support tissue
2. Common in the elderly
3. Purpuric lesions—common on the dorsum of the hand (loose
   skin)
4. No effective treatment (but exclude e.g. scurvy)

DRUG/INFECTION INDUCED PURPURA

A variety of drugs and many infections may sometimes cause
vasculitic reactions.

HYPERCORTICOSTEROIDISM

In Cushing's disease or as a result of corticosteroid therapy – due to
atrophy of skin and subcutaneous tissue.

DERANGED SERUM BIOCHEMISTRY

Uraemia and dysproteinaemias.

PLATELET DISORDERS

1. Failure of adequate platelet production:
   (i)   Hereditary thrombocytopenias, e.g. Wiskott–Aldrich
         syndrome (eczema, thrombocytopenia plus impaired cellular
         and humoral immunity), TAR syndrome (thrombocytopenia
         with absent radii). Bernard Soulier syndrome (giant platelets
         and thrombocytopenia)
   (ii) Megakaryocytes reduced in number, e.g. aplastic anaemia or
         marrow infiltration
   (iii) Platelet formation defective, e.g. ineffective

thrombocytopoiesis in megaloblastic anaemias, alcohol abuse
2. Increased loss of platelets in circulation due to:
   (i)   Destruction of immunologically sensitised platelets—chiefly in the spleen (most forms of ITP)
   (ii) Splenic pooling ('hypersplenism')
   (iii) Consumption in intravascular coagulopathies
   (iv) Massive or exchange transfusion

IDIOPATHIC THROMBOCYTOPENIC PURPURA (ITP)

Aetiology
The majority of cases are probably autoimmune but may be 'triggered' by e.g. viral infections.

Haematology
1. Anaemia, when it occurs, is secondary to haemorrhagic complications. The indices may reflect iron deficiency
2. WBC—may be increased during bleeds
3. Platelets – decreased, sometimes $< 10 \times 10^9$/l. Platelet antibodies are detectable in 80% of cases
4. Bone marrow—typically, megakaryocytes *increased* in number; they often appear immature with sharply demarcated cytoplasm and no platelet budding
5. Prolonged bleeding time, using standardised template method

Clinical features
1. May occur at any age but is commoner in children and young adults. Post-puberty, there is a female preponderance
2. Onset—can be explosive (especially in children) or insidious
3. Bleeding, spontaneous or post-traumatic, at various sites:
   (i)   Skin—petechiae and ecchymoses
   (ii) Mucous membranes—e.g. epistaxis, bleeding gums
   (iii) Menorrhagia; haematuria; melaena
   (iv) CNS bleeds—may be fatal. Retinal haemorrhages (indicator of severity)
4. Physical signs relate to the bleeding complications Splenomegaly is not usual; seen more commonly in children

Clinical types

1. Acute
(i)   Often in children and post-infective
(ii) Commonly self-limiting with spontaneous resolution
(iii) Most severe at onset

2. Sub-acute/chronic
(i)   Usually in adults

(ii) Often persistent but fluctuating symptoms with variable 'remissions'

Treatment

1. Of acute ITP
(i) Observation (mild cases) and avoidance of injury
(ii) Corticosteroids (e.g. prednisolone 60 mg daily)— often produce rapid symptomatic response and hasten spontaneous remission
(iii) Intravenous immunoglobulins—usual alternative to steroids to produce rapid increase in platelet count
(iv) Platelet transfusions—for severe life-threatening thrombocytopenia, but rarely indicated

2. Of sub-acute/chronic ITP
Persisting, symptomatic, moderate to severe thrombocytopenia requires concerted management:
(i) Corticosteroids—the first-line treatment, but suboptimal response within 3 weeks is an indication to proceed to alternatives
(ii) Splenectomy—often indicated if early response to corticosteroids is inadequate or platelet count falls as steroid dosage is reduced. The principal disadvantage of splenectomy is the susceptibility of splenectomised patients to infection (especially children, in whom a longer trial of steroids is usually indicated). Prophylactic pneumococcal vaccine pre-splenectomy and penicillin V post-splenectomy indicated
Overall, steroid therapy ± splenectomy results in 75% complete or good partial remissions.
(iii) Intravenous immunoglobulin (0.4 g/kg daily for 5 days or 0.7 g/kg daily for 3 days):
   a. Causes rapid, but transient improvement in 70% of cases (by reticulo-endothelial blockade)
   b. Useful method of boosting platelet count to cover elective surgery and episodes of life-threatening bleeding in chronic ITP
   c. Treatment of choice for ITP of late pregnancy, where steroids and cytotoxic agents are contraindicated
(iv) Cytotoxic drugs (for probable immunosuppressive effects) e.g. azathioprine, cyclophosphamide, vincristine and danazol (an androgen) may be of value in the refractory splenectomised patient
(v) Supportive—red cell and platelet transfusions (of limited value due to reduced platelet survival time).
Intramuscular injections and antiplatelet drugs should be avoided

Course and prognosis

Varies considerably with type and age. Optimal survival depends on careful management. CNS bleeding is the commonest cause of death (< 5% cases of chronic ITP, < 1% of acute ITP).

OTHER IMMUNE THROMBOCYTOPENIAS (some are labelled ITP)

Associations

1. Antibodies to the platelet antigen PL^{A1} cause post-transfusion purpura in previously sensitised multiparous females, and isoimmune neonatal thrombocytopenia in PL^{A1}-positive infants born to PL^{A1}-negative (previously sensitised) mothers
2. Haematological malignancies, e.g. lymphomas
3. Collagen disease, notably SLE (very important in the differential diagnosis of ITP)
4. Infections—e.g. rubella, infectious mononucleosis
5. Drug ingestion:
   (i) immune-complex-mediated, e.g. quinine, quinidine
   (ii) platelet aggregation, e.g. heparin, ristocetin

Treatment

1. Of the primary disease or withdrawal of drug
2. Corticosteroids may be of value (in 2–4 above)
3. For neonatal isoimmune thrombocytopenia, transfusion of PL^{A1}-negative platelets ± i.v. immunoglobulins

THROMBOTIC THROMBOCYTOPENIAS

1. Haemolytic uraemic syndrome (HUS)
2. Thrombotic thrombocytopenic purpura (TTP)
3. Disseminated intravascular coagulation (DIC)—see p.141

HUS/TTP

There is good evidence that HUS and TTP represent the same disease process with different distribution of thrombotic lesions.

Aetiology

1. Infective—e.g. diarrhoeal prodrome in epidemic HUS, verotoxin
2. Prostacyclin deficiency ± absence of prostacyclin stimulatory factor
3. Spontaneous platelet aggregation due to deficiency of an IgG inhibitor of a platelet aggregatory factor in normal plasma
4. Excess of high molecular weight multimers of von Willebrand's factor, causing platelet adhesion to vascular endothelium

Pathology
Endothelial swelling in capillaries and precapillary arterioles with platelet adhesion, aggregation and release, and fibrin deposition.

Haematology
1. Microangiopathic haemolytic anaemia with RBC fragments and schistocytes on film
2. Thrombocytopenia
3. Normal or slightly prolonged PT, APTT, and TT (cf. DIC)
4. Normal fibrinogen; FDPs may be slightly raised

HUS

Clinical features
1. Epidemic—acute onset, often preceded by diarrhoeal illness in young children
2. Sporadic—insidious, often familial. Poor prognosis
3. Acute renal failure
4. Hypertension

Treatment
1. Dialysis
2. Control of hypertension
3. RBC transfusions
4. Plasma infusions
5. Plasma exchange

Prognosis
5–30% mortality. Worst with familial relapsing disease
One-third recover fully
One-third have persistent hypertension ± chronic renal impairment
One-third have persistent oliguric acute renal failure

TTP

Clinical features
1. Slight female preponderance; peak incidence 30–40 years
2. Majority of cases are idiopathic. May be related to pregnancy, autoimmune disease or drug-induced (e.g. cyclosporin A, oral contraceptives)
3. Fever
4. Fluctuating neurological abnormalities—confusion, coma, convulsions
5. Progressive renal impairment

Treatment
As for HUS, with broad-spectrum antibiotics. Antiplatelet agents may be of some benefit.

Prognosis
Worse than for HUS. Mortality ≈ 50%.

DISORDERS OF PLATELET FUNCTION

1. Congenital
(i)   Connective tissue disorders, e.g. Ehlers-Danlos
(ii) Plasma protein disorders, e.g. afibrinogenaemia
⎫ cause secondary
⎬ platelet dysfunction
⎭
(iii) Primary platelet defects—see Table 16.1

Table 16.1   Primary platelet defects — aggregation studies

Disorder	ADP	Adrenaline	Collagen	Ristocetin	Arachidonic acid	Bovine fibrinogen
Bernard –Soulier syndrome (GPIb deficiency)	N	N	N	–	N	Abnormal
Thromboasthenia (Glanzmann's) GPIIb/IIIa deficiency	–	–	–	N	–	–
Storage pool defect	No second phase	No second phase	↓	N	N	
von Willebrand's	N	N	N	–	N	N

N = normal, – = absent, ↓ = reduced

2. Acquired
(i)   Drug-induced—e.g. acetylsalicylic acid (aspirin) inhibits cycloxygenase activity, resulting in normal aggregation with ADP and ristocetin, but abnormal with adrenaline, collagen and arachidonic acid (effects of 300 mg last up to 7 days). Indomethacin and phenylbutazone generally have short-lived effects.

(ii) Myeloproliferative disorders, e.g. thrombocythaemia
(iii) Myelodysplasia
(iv) Renal disease—uraemia, nephrotic syndrome
(v) Dysproteinaemia—Waldenström's macroglobulinaemia, myeloma

COAGULATION FACTOR DEFICIENCIES

Basic physiology
Normal coagulation results from activation of pro-enzymes (circulating inactive precursors of the clotting factors)—see Figure 16.1 and Table 16.2.

Classification
1. Congenital—hereditary deficiencies of each of the coagulation proteins have been recorded
2. Acquired—due to:
   (i) Vitamin K deficiency
   (ii) Liver disease
   (iii) Consumption coagulopathy
   (iv) Circulating inhibitors

HAEMOPHILIA A (Factor VIII deficiency)

The Factor VIII molecule consists of:
1. FVIII—coagulant protein defective in haemophilia A

Table 16.2 Screening tests for detecting coagulation factor deficiencies

Factor deficiency	PT	APTT/KCCT	Bleeding time
I	↑	↑	N
II	↑	↑	N
V	↑	↑	N or ↑
VII	↑	N	N
VIII Haemophilia A	N	↑	N
VIII vWD	N	↑	N or ↑
IX	N	↑	N
X	↑	↑	N
XI	N	↑	N
XII	N	↑	N
XIII	N	N	N

N = Normal   ↑ = Increased

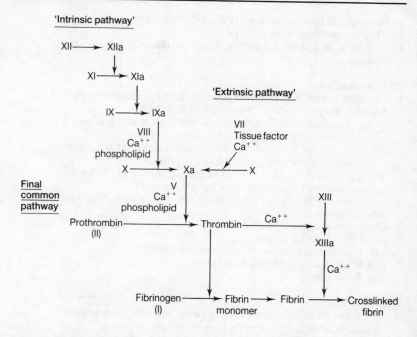

'Intrinsic pathway'

'Extrinsic pathway'

Final common pathway

Prothrombin time (PT) measures extrinsic and final common pathways
Activated partial thromboplastin time (APTT) or Kaolin cephalin clotting time (KCCT)
measure intrinsic and final common pathways

Fig. 16.1 The coagulation cascade

2. Von Willebrand's factor (vWF)—glycoprotein carrier for
   coagulant protein. Defective in von Willebrand's disease.
   Measured functionally by ristocetin cofactor activity (RiCoF)
3. Von Willebrand's factor antigen (vWFAg)—immunological
   determinant of vWF

Genetics
Sex-linked recessive transmission.
  Incidence—1:10 000 population; 25% cases are spontaneous
mutations

Pathology
1. Synthesis of abnormal factor VIII molecules
2. Decreased coagulant activity

Haematology
1. Prolonged partial thromboplastin time (APTT)

2. Plasma VIII low or absent; vWF and vWFAg normal
3. PT and bleeding time normal
4. Anaemia, if it occurs, has the features of blood loss, acute or chronic

Clinical features
1. Variable (patient to patient) susceptibility to spontaneous haemorrhage. Tends to 'run true' in families
   (i) VIII activity < 1%—severe bleeds after trivial trauma; spontaneous bleeds into muscles and joints
   (ii) VIII activity 1–5%—moderate to severe post-traumatic bleeds; occasional spontaneous bleeds
   (iii) VIII activity 5–25%—mild bleeding tendency, though excessive blood loss may follow surgery
2. Variable intensity of symptoms in the individual. Improvement after puberty
3. Common bleeds:
   (i) Into synovial joints
   (ii) Into muscle (especially in severe cases)
   (iii) From gums and tooth sockets
   (iv) Epistaxis

Complications
1. Arthritis—usually secondary to recurrent haemorrhages
2. Pressure effects of haematomas—peripheral nerve compression, pseudotumours
3. FVIII antibodies/inhibitors—in 5–10% patients, related to previous treatment. More common in severe haemophilia
4. Chronic liver disease—chronically raised transaminase levels seen in 70% haemophiliacs. May herald chronic persistent or chronic active hepatitis. Related to previous exposure to hepatitis B or C.
5. Acquired immunodeficiency syndrome (AIDS)—due to retroviral contamination of FVIII concentrates in the early 1980s. All concentrates are now heat-treated and from an HIV-negative donor pool in UK. Kaposi's sarcoma is extremely rare in haemophilia-related AIDS

Treatment
1. Prophylaxis:
   (i) Avoidance of trauma
   (ii) Administration of factor VIII concentrates, cryoprecipitate, DDAVP, e.g. before surgical procedures DDAVP (deamino-8-D-arginine vasopressin) is given by i.v. (0.3 µg/kg) or intranasal (2 µg/kg) routes and increases FVIII levels by mobilising tissue stores in mild haemophiliacs, avoiding the need for blood products. Stimulates release of vascular plasminogen activator, so should be

used with tranexamic acid to inhibit the fibrinolytic stimulus
2. Of bleeding—factor VIII concentrates (heat-treated) now considered preferable to cryoprecipitate (not heat-treated). Recombinant FVIII should be commercially available by mid-1990s. Tranexamic acid may be beneficial. Early home treatment (where possible) reduces severity of bleeding
3. Of factor VIII inhibitors:
   (i)   Porcine factor VIII
   (ii) FEIBA (factor VIII inhibitor bypassing activity)—an activated complex of uncertain mechanism of action
   (iii) Activated factor VII
   (iv) Steroids ± immunosuppressive therapy
   (v)   Plasma exchange
4. Of chronic liver disease—α interferon may be beneficial. Trials are in progress
5. Of AIDS—counselling and contraceptive advice; prophylaxis against *Pneumocystis* pneumonia with nebulised pentamidine

The modern treatment of haemophilia involves multidisciplinary teams including haematologists, nurses, dentists, orthopaedic surgeons, physiotherapists, social workers and genetic counsellors.

HAEMOPHILIA B (or 'Christmas disease'—named after a patient)

Genetics
Sex-linked recessive transmission. Less frequent than haemophilia A (1:50 000).

Pathology
Defective factor IX production.

Haematology
Essentially as for haemophilia A but with low plasma factor IX activity.

Clinical features
Essentially as for haemophilia A.

Treatment
1. General principles as for haemophilia A
2. FIX concentrates—higher doses initially required because of low recovery; $t_{\frac{1}{2}}$ = 18 hours so daily infusions adequate subsequently
3. Development of inhibitors is less frequent than in haemophilia A (1% cases)

VON WILLEBRAND'S DISEASE

Numerous subtypes (IA–C, IIA–F, III) are distinguishable by multimeric analysis and using gene probes.

Genetics
Autosomal dominant transmission.

Pathology
1. Decreased Factor VIII coagulant protein (FVIII) production
2. Deficient vWF glycoprotein carrier, causing defective platelet adhesion to subendothelium

Haematology
1. Prolonged APTT/KCCT and bleeding time
2. Low or absent vWF
3. Low FVIII and vWFAg
4. Defective platelet aggregation in response to ristocetin
5. Anaemia, if it occurs, has features of blood loss—acute/chronic

Clinical features
1. Family history of bleeding tendency
2. Abnormal bleeding from mucosal surfaces (gums, epistaxis, menorrhagia) and small cuts. Joint bleeds uncommon

Treatment
Depends on site and severity of bleeding:
1. DDAVP—effective in mild or moderate bleeding in type I and most type II subgroups. Contraindicated in type IIB—may precipitate thrombocytopenia by inducing platelet aggregation in vivo
2. Cryoprecipitate—severe type I and most type II subgroups. Risk of viral disease transmission, but a more effective source of vWF than highly purified FVIII concentrates. Bleeding time corrected for 12 hours but FVIII level peaks 12–24 hours after treatment
3. Factor VIII concentrates—less risk of infection than with cryoprecipitate, but may not be as effective as vWF content lower. Current UK recommendations state that VIII concentrates should be used initially and cryoprecipitate only if haemostasis not achieved with concentrates
4. Oestrogens and antifibrinolytics may control menorrhagia

ACQUIRED COAGULATION DISEASES

HAEMORRHAGIC DISEASE OF THE NEWBORN ('PRIMARY')

Aetiology
1. Reduced stores of vitamin K   ⎫ especially in
2. Reduced synthetic capacity of the liver ⎭ premature infants

Pathology
Impaired synthesis of prothrombin and factors VII, IX and X.

Haematology
1. Indices—normal or reflect blood loss
2. Platelets—normal
3. Blood film—polychromasia, increased normoblasts
4. Prothrombin time—prolonged
5. PIVKA II (protein induced by vitamin K absence) positive

Clinical features
1. Association with poor socioeconomic conditions
2. More frequent in breast-fed infants (cows' milk contains 4×
   vitamin K content)
3. Haemorrhages—usually occur on 2nd–4th day of life, at various
   sites, e.g. scalp, umbilicus, gastrointestinal tract, circumcision
   site, intraventricular

Treatment
1. Specific—parenteral administration of vitamin K (which may
   also be given prophylactically—1 mg)
2. Supportive—blood, fresh frozen plasma (more rapidly effective
   than vitamin K)

MALABSORPTION OF VITAMIN K

Minimal daily requirement is 0.1–0.5 µg/kg.

Causes
1. Biliary obstruction (lack of bile salts)
2. Adult coeliac disease, sprue
3. Gut sterilisation (altered flora)
4. Small intestinal resection

Pathology
Impaired synthesis of prothrombin and factors VII, IX and X, protein
S and protein C.

Haematology
1. Features of blood loss (acute/chronic) may be present

2. Features of the associated disease, e.g. megaloblastosis
3. Prothrombin time—prolonged

Clinical features
1. Haemorrhagic tendency – the type of bleeding resembling that in haemophilia, usually mild
2. Of the associated disease

Treatment
1. Of the associated disease
2. Parenteral vitamin K if necessary for bleeds

VITAMIN K ANTAGONISTS

1. Oral anticoagulants, e.g. warfarin
2. Some cephalosporins, e.g. cephamandole

LIVER DISEASE

Pathogenesis
Multifactorial:
1. Impaired synthesis of prothrombin and factors VII, IX and X (vitamin K-dependent)
2. Impaired synthesis of factors V and fibrinogen (severe hepatic damage and dysfibrinogenaemia)
3. Thrombocytopenia—due to folate depletion, alcoholism and/ or hypersplenism
4. Fibrinolysis

Haematology
As for Vitamin K deficiency but with additional clotting defects, evidence of folate deficiency

Clinical features
Haemorrhagic tendency—usually mild, though severe bleeds may occur from varices and in end-stage liver failure

Treatment
1. Of the primary disease
2. Vitamin K (which alone may be relatively ineffective) ± fresh frozen plasma
3. Folic acid may be indicated

DISSEMINATED INTRAVASCULAR COAGULATION

Occurs in a wide range of clinical situations.

Definition
Reduction in circulating clotting factors due to intravascular thromboses initiated by a variety of events

Pathogenesis
1. Release of thromboplastic substances into the circulation and activation of the extrinsic clotting system:
   (i)   Following surgical trauma
   (ii) Consequent to obstetric complications, e.g. placental separation, retained dead fetus, amniotic fluid embolism
   (iii) In acute haemolytic episodes
   (iv) In malignancy, e.g. due to tumour necrosis
2. Activation of the intrinsic clotting system
3. Induction of platelet aggregation
4. Deposition of fibrin in small blood vessels with local ischaemic changes (e.g. in kidney)
5. Secondary activation of fibrinolysis—breakdown of fibrin with production of fibrin degradation products (FDP)
6. Consumption of clotting factors and platelets. Coagulopathy

Haematology
1. Thrombocytopenia
2. Blood film—red cell fragments and schistocytes
3. Bleeding and prothrombin times, APTT and TT—prolonged
4. Fibrinogen level—decreased. Fibrin degradation products (FDP) and D-dimers present
5. Factors V and VIII—low

These findings are not invariable—the *degree* of consumption coagulopathy varies. The platelet count, blood film, FDP assay and thrombin time together are the most helpful in diagnosis

Clinical features
1. Some patients are asymptomatic
2. Symptoms and signs relating to associated disease (see below)
3. Symptoms and signs relating to DIC per se
   (i)   Haemorrhagic manifestations of variable severity (due to consumption coagulopathy)
   (ii) 'Microangiopathic' haemolytic anaemia (due to red cell distortion/fragmentation in small blood vessels)
   (iii) Renal/adrenal failure due to intravascular thrombosis)

Associations
1. Severe infection, e.g. Gram-negative septicaemia (60% cases)
2. Malignant disease—metastatic carcinomas, (especially of lung, stomach, pancreas, prostate), promyelocytic leukaemia
3. Trauma—surgery, obstetric accidents
4. Burns
5. Antigen–antibody reactions, e.g. severe immune haemolysis

Treatment
1. Of the underlying disease/precipitating factor—e.g. antibiotics in septicaemia
2. Heparin—sometimes of value but indiscriminate use is dangerous
3. Blood products—may aggravate; correct timing and great care is necessary
4. Tranexamic acid—antifibrinolytic activity can be helpful in some cases

CIRCULATING INHIBITORS

Development of anticoagulants/inhibitors directed against clotting factors, notably VIII.
1. Idiopathic
2. In association with collagen disease, e.g. SLE, RA
3. In haemophilia A (anti-factor VIII)—seen in 5–10% patients
4. 'Lupus anticoagulant'—antiphospholipid antibody which inhibits normal coagulation cascade. Associated with prolonged APTT and positive anticardiolipin antibodies. Clinically associated with *thrombotic* tendency, recurrent abortions and placental dysfunction. Treated with steroids, anticoagulants and/or aspirin.

FURTHER ADVANCED READING

Poller L (ed) 1991 Recent advances in blood coagulation 5. Churchill Livingstone, Edinburgh
Thomson J M 1991 Blood coagulation and haemostasis. 4th edn, Churchill Livingstone, Edinburgh

17. Thrombosis and anticoagulation

THROMBOSIS

Thrombosis (arterial or venous) results from combinations of the following factors:
1. Vascular endothelial damage
2. Altered blood flow
3. Altered platelet activity
4. Imbalance between coagulation/fibrinolytic pathways

ARTERIAL THROMBOSIS

Pathogenesis

Atheromatous endothelial damage with platelet adhesion and fibrin generation. Relative imbalance between generation of proaggregatory thromboxane A_2 and antiaggregatory prostacyclin may favour thrombosis.

Associations
1. Hypertension
2. Atherosclerosis
3. Hyperlipidaemia
4. Diabetes mellitus
5. Polycythaemia
6. Gout
7. Smoking
8. Familial (see below)

Clinical features
1. ± history of intermittent claudication
2. Ischaemic pain
3. Distal pallor → cyanosis → gangrene
4. Absent distal pulsation

Diagnosis
1. Clinical assessment
2. Angiography

VENOUS THROMBOSIS

Pathogenesis
Excessive local thrombin production (with fibrin deposition and platelet aggregation) in vessels with low flow rates without underlying vascular endothelial damage.

Associations
1. Immobilisation—postoperative, CVAs
2. Trauma, especially fractured neck of femur
3. Obesity
4. Pregnancy
5. Myeloproliferative disorders
6. Carcinoma (± thrombophlebitis migrans)
7. Drugs—oral contraceptives, steroids, asparaginase
8. Lupus anticoagulant (antiphospholipid antibody)
9. Behçet's syndrome
10. Central venous cannulae, e.g. Hickman line
11. Familial (see below)
12. Miscellaneous abnormalities of clotting systems, e.g. dysfibrinogenaemia, plasminogen deficiency, tissue plasminogen activator inhibitor (TPAI), heparin cofactor II deficiency

Clinical features
1. Localised warmth and tenderness
2. Swelling
3. Peripheral vasodilatation due to opening up of collateral circulation
4. Positive Homan's sign (unreliable)

Diagnosis
1. Venography
2. Impedance plethysmography
3. Doppler ultrasonography

FAMILIAL THROMBOTIC DISORDERS

Protein C deficiency (normal range 0.61—1.32 u/ml)
1. Autosomal dominant transmission with variable penetrance
2. Deficiency of a vitamin-K-dependent protein which has anticoagulant activity by inhibition of Va and VIIIa and stimulation of fibrinolysis
3. Subtypes:
    (i) Type I—reduced PC activity and reduced PC antigen
    (ii) Type II—reduced PC activity and normal PC antigen

4. Causes 5–8% of venous thromboses in patients under 40 years
5. Homozygous forms cause purpura fulminans at birth
6. Less severe forms associated with warfarin-induced skin necrosis. Such patients should be heparinised before introducing warfarin
7. Acquired deficiency seen in liver disease, DIC and warfarin therapy

Protein S deficiency (normal ranges total PS 0.67–1.25 u/ml and free PS 0.23–0.49 u/ml)

1. Autosomal dominant transmission
2. Deficiency of a vitamin-K-dependent protein, which acts as cofactor for protein C

Antithrombin III (ATIII) deficiency

1. Autosomal dominant transmission
2. Deficiency of ATIII which normally inactivates XIIa, XIa, IXa, Xa, thrombin and plasmin. ATIII is required for the action of heparin
3. Sub-types:
   - (i) Type I—reduced biological activity and reduced ATIII antigen
   - (ii) Type II—reduced biological activity and normal ATIII antigen
4. Causes 2–4% of venous thromboses in patients under 30 years
5. Acquired deficiency seen in liver disease, nephrotic syndrome, DIC and oral contraceptive therapy
6. ATIII concentrates may be required in the treatment of DIC and acute thrombosis (rarely)

ANTICOAGULATION

HEPARIN

Naturally occurring glycosaminoglycan (mol. wt 15 000—18 000). Low molecular weight heparins (mol. wt 5 000) now commercially available.

1. Action
- (i) Binds with ATIII, potentiating its inhibitory action on thrombin, XIIa, XIa, IXa, and Xa
- (ii) Low molecular weight heparins have more specific anti-Xa activity, longer $T_{\frac{1}{2}}$ (twice that of standard heparin) and less platelet interaction
- (iii) Does not cross placenta
- (iv) Immediate action after intravenous administration

2. Indications
- (i) Early treatment of acute thrombosis

(ii)   Treatment and prophylaxis of thrombosis in pregnancy
(iii) Surgical prophylaxis in high-risk situations, e.g. pelvic surgery

3. Treatment regimens
Lower doses are required to inhibit thrombin formation rather than
to neutralise formed thrombin; prophylactic doses are therefore
lower than therapeutic doses:
(i)   Subcutaneous, e.g. 5000 units unfractionated heparin 8–12-
      hourly or 2000–5000 units low molecular weight heparin daily
      for surgical prophylaxis and in pregnancy
(ii) Intravenous, e.g. 10 000 units 6-hourly by continuous infusion
      for acute thrombosis. Treatment should be continued after
      introduction of oral anticoagulants until therapeutic INR
      achieved (see below)

4. Monitoring
(i)   Monitoring not required for 'low-dose' prophylaxis and
      subcutaneous treatment regimes
(ii) Monitor i.v. treatment using APTT or KCCT (measures intrinsic
      pathway)
(iii) Therapeutic range = 2–2.5×normal

5. Treatment of overdosage
(i)   Discontinue heparin—usually rapid effect because of short
      intravenous $t_{\frac{1}{2}}$ (30–120 min); monitor APTT/KCCT and clinical
      state
(ii) Protamine sulphate (1 mg i.v. neutralises 100 u heparin). Not
      indicated in the absence of bleeding; excess protamine can
      cause haemorrhagic and allergic reactions

6. Side effects
(i)   Bleeding
(ii) Osteoporosis—rare; associated with long-term therapy
(iii) Thrombocytopenia—immune-mediated; secondary platelet
      dysfunction

ORAL ANTICOAGULANTS
Coumarins, particularly warfarin, most commonly used.

Warfarin

1. Action
(i)   Inhibits vitamin-K-dependent hepatic gamma-carboxylation of
      glutamic acid residues of II, VII, IX and X necessary to allow
      binding of calcium and phospholipid in the coagulation
      sequence
(ii) Inhibits actions of proteins C and S

(iii) Due to variation in $t_{\frac{1}{2}}$ of II, VII, IX and X it takes 48–72 hours to obtain full anticoagulant effect. Protein C and VII levels fall first ($t_{\frac{1}{2}} = 6$ h) and can be associated with a transient prothrombotic state (due to secondary protein C deficiency) if patient is not heparinised

(iv) Crosses placenta and excreted in small (safe) quantities in breast milk. Contraindicated in early pregnancy and labour (see below)

(v) $T_{\frac{1}{2}}$ approximately 40 hours

(vi) Interaction with other drugs—anticoagulant effect may be increased or reduced:
   a. Increased—e.g. by alcohol, penicillin, NSAIDs, oral hypoglycaemics, quinine, laxatives, aspirin (also has antiplatelet effect)
   b. Reduced—e.g. by barbiturates, phenytoin, spironolactone, oral contraceptives

2. Indications
Prophylaxis and treatment of thrombotic disorders

3. Treatment regimen and duration
(i) If baseline PT and liver function tests are normal, initial dosage is warfarin 10 mg on day 1, 10 mg on day 2 and 5 mg on day 3, at a fixed time

(ii) Maintenance dose usually 3-9 mg/d with wide individual variations depending on concurrent medications, compliance

(iii) Patient should be given clearly written dosage instructions and should be advised of possible complications

(iv) Duration of treatment depends on underlying condition:
   a. Single DVT—3 months ⎫
   b. Pulmonary embolism   ⎬ 3–6 months
   c. Myocardial infarction ⎭
   d. Recurrent thromboembolism ⎫
   e. Prosthetic heart valves   ⎪
   f. PC/PS/ATIII deficiency with recurrent thrombosis ⎬ long-term
   g. Lupus anticoagulant with thrombosis ⎭

4. Monitoring
(i) Close monitoring required initially until stabilisation of anticoagulation. Stable patients need checks about every 2 months in an anticoagulant clinic

(ii) Treatment is monitored by the International Normalised Ratio (INR). This is derived from the PT and standardises results despite variation in thromboplastin sensitivities for different PT test methods

(iii) Recommended INR depends on underlying condition (Haemostasis and Thrombosis Task Force criteria):
   a. 2.0–2.5—DVT prophylaxis for high risk surgery

b. 2.0–3.0—DVT prophylaxis for hip surgery and fractured femur. Treatment of DVT/pulmonary embolism. Transient ischaemic attacks. Atrial fibrillation
c. 3.0–4.5—Recurrent DVT and pulmonary embolism. Arterial disease including myocardial infarction. Prosthetic heart valves and grafts

5. Treatment of overdosage
Depends on severity of bleeding, patient's ability to tolerate fluid loads, risk of viral transmission with blood products and possible thrombotic risks of overcorrection with vitamin K:
(i) INR > 4.5 without haemorrhage—withold warfarin for a few days and monitor
(ii) INR > 4.5 with minor bleeding—withold warfarin; ± vitamin K 2.5 mg i.v.
(iii) INR > 4.5 with life-threatening bleeding – withold warfarin; vitamin K 5–10 mg i.v.; fresh frozen plasma (2–4 units) and monitor
Fresh frozen plasma gives rapid controlled correction; vitamin K may take 6 hours for full response and larger doses may make patient refractory to oral anticoagulants for weeks
(iv) INR in therapeutic range with excessive bleeding—exclude previously unsuspected pathology (e.g. renal or gastrointestinal)

6. Side effects
(i) Bleeding
(ii) Teratogenicity—crosses placenta and can cause retroplacental and fetal intracranial haemorrhage, blindness, microcephaly, mental retardation, saddle nose and chondrodysplasia
(iii) 'Purple foot' syndrome—discoloured, sometimes gangrenous skin patches associated with early warfarin treatment; due to primary or secondary protein C deficiency

FIBRINOLYTICS
1. 'First-generation' agents:
   Streptokinase, urokinase
2. 'Second-generation' agents:
   (i) Tissue plasminogen activator (rtPA), single chain urokinase plasminogen activator (scuPA)
   (ii) Anisoylatedlys-plasminogen-streptokinase, activator complex (APSAC—anistreplase)

1. Action
(i) Direct or indirect activation of plasminogen, with stimulation of the fibrinolytic pathway (Fig. 17.1)

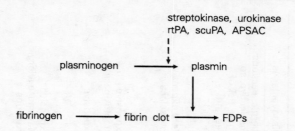

Fig. 17.1

(ii) Remove intravascular fibrin clot by lysis, preserving vascular patency (cf. conventional anticoagulants, which only prevent further clot propagation)
(iii) Selectivity of drug for fibrin-bound rather than free plasminogen affects degree of systemic defibrination; first-generation drugs are *less* selective and are associated with more severe bleeding complications

2. Indications
(i) Massive pulmonary embolism
(ii) Acute myocardial infarction—several multicentre trials confirm a 20–50% reduction in mortality if thrombolytic therapy given within 4–6 hours of onset of symptoms
(iii) Acute peripheral vascular occlusion (if surgery contraindicated)

3. Treatment regimes. (see Table 17.1)
There is some evidence of synergism with rtPA + scuPA and rtPA + urokinase combination therapy

4. Monitoring
(i) Close clinical assessment essential
(ii) Laboratory monitoring not required for short duration treatment
(iii) For prolonged treatment, monitor using the thrombin time; therapeutic range = 3–5×normal

5. Treatment of overdosage
(i) In view of relatively short $t_{\frac{1}{2}}$s of fibrinolytic agents, discontinuing treatment alone is usually adequate
(ii) Antifibrinolytic agents, e.g. tranexamic acid, effective for treatment of life-threatening bleeding

6. Side effects
(i) Bleeding (30% of patients overall):
    a. commonly at sites of i.v. cannulation
    b. major in 10% cases; life threatening in < 1% cases

Table 17.1 Fibrinolytic agents

Fibrinolytic agent	Source	$t_\frac{1}{2}$	Recommended dose	Advantages	Disadvantages
Streptokinase	β-haemolytic streptococci	20 min	Acute MI: 1 500 000 u i.v. over 1 h; Massive PE: 250 000 u i.v. over 30 min, then 100 000 u i.v. hourly for 12–48 h (then standard anticoagulation)	Inexpensive	Allergic reactions Unselective, so higher risk of bleeding
Urokinase	Human urine and fetal kidney cells	16 min	Acute MI: 2 000 000 u i.v. over 1 h; PE: 300 000 u i.v. over 30 min, then 300 000 u i.v. hourly for 12–48 h	Not allergenic	More expensive Low selectivity
Recombinant tissue plasminogen (rtPA)	Recombinant DNA technology	5–8 min	Acute MI: 100 mg i.v. over 3 h	More selective	Expensive (10 × streptokinase)
Single chain plasminogen (scuPA)	Recombinant DNA technology	5–8 min	Acute MI: 50–70 mg i.v. over 1 h	More selective Fewer bleeding problems	Expensive
Acylated plasminogen streptokinase activated complex (APSAC, anistreplase)		90 min	Acute MI: 30 u i.v. over 5 min	Highly selective Very few bleeding problems	Expensive May cause allergic reactions

   c. generally more common with first-generation agents, but ISIS-3 and GISSI-2 trials showed a highly significant increase in cerebral haemorrhage with rtPA

(ii) Allergic reactions—fever, antibody formation with streptokinase and APSAC (less commonly)

(iii) Nausea and vomiting

(iv) Re-perfusion arrhythmias

7. Contraindications
Patients with previous history of:
(i)   Peptic ulceration
(ii) Recent surgery (within 6 weeks)
(iii) Recent CVA
(iv) Severe hypertension
(v) Recent streptococcal infection or streptokinase treatment within last 6 months (streptokinase only)

ANCROD

1. Proteolytic polypeptide derived from viper venom
2. Cleaves fibrinopeptide A from fibrinogen, preventing normal cross-linkage during polymerisation. Produces a friable fibrin clot very susceptible to lysis by plasmin
3. Causes profound hypofibrinogenaemia, but rarely serious bleeding problems
4. Similar efficacy to heparin in DVT prevention, but rarely used
5. Hypersensitivity quite common

ANTIPLATELET DRUGS

Rationale for their use is based on the rôle of platelets in aetiology of arterial thrombosis (see p.143).

Aspirin
1. Inactivates cyclo-oxygenase:
   (i)   In platelets (low dose) preventing synthesis of thromboxane A_2 (proaggregatory vasoconstrictor)
   (ii) In endothelium (standard doses) preventing synthesis of prostacyclin (antiaggregatory vasodilator)
2. Use of low-dose aspirin (75 mg daily or alternate days) should favour a more selective antithromboxane A_2 effect
3. Of proven benefit in the treatment of:
   (i)   Digital ischaemia in myeloproliferative disorders associated with thrombocytosis
   (ii) Transient rebound thrombocytosis following splenectomy
   (iii) Transient ischaemic attacks
   (iv) Patients following coronary artery bypass graft surgery (CABG)

Dipyridamole
1. Inhibits phosphodiesterase, increasing inhibitory levels of platelet cyclic AMP and possibly potentiating effect of prostacyclin
2. Of no definite benefit as antithrombotic agent

Sulphinpyrazole
1. Uricosuric agent, interfering with platelet function by ill-defined action
2. Beneficial in treatment of patients following CABG

FURTHER ADVANCED READING

Collen D, Stump D C, Gold H K 1988 Thrombolytic therapy. In: Hoffbrand A V (ed) Recent advances in haematology 5. Churchill Livingstone, Edinburgh, pp 265–274

Hirsh J (ed) 1990 Antithrombotic therapy. Clinical haematology 3:3. Baillière Tindall, London

Roberts B E (ed) 1991 Investigation and management of thrombophilia. In: Standard haematology practice. Blackwell, Oxford, pp 112–127

Roberts B E (ed) 1991 Oral anticoagulation. In: Standard haematology practice. Blackwell, Oxford, pp 73–87

18. Blood products

The development of blood component therapy as an alternative to whole blood transfusion allows more efficient utilisation of a finite blood supply, with increased availability of plasma for fractionation into FVIII and IX concentrates and immunoglobulins (normal and hyperimmune).

RED CELLS

Basic concepts

1. Erythrocytes contain genetically determined cell membrane antigens. Many blood group systems have been defined; two are of major importance:
   (i)   ABO
   (ii) Rhesus (especially D)
2. Antibodies to the antigens are of two types:
   (i)   Naturally occurring (i.e. without obvious stimulation), e.g. anti-B agglutinins in persons with group A red cells
   (ii) Immune—resulting from antigenic stimulus, e.g. rhesus antibodies produced by transfusion of Rh +ve cells into Rh −ve person, or following fetomaternal haemorrhage
3. Antibodies can also be classified as:
   (i)   Complete—agglutination of red cells bearing corresponding antigen seen in saline (most naturally occurring types, typically IgM)
   (ii) Incomplete—agglutination of red cells bearing corresponding antigen seen in enzyme or macromolecular media, e.g. albumin (most immune types, typically, IgG). Demonstrable by indirect Coombs test
4. Immune anti-A and anti-B antibodies result from:
   (i)   Previous incompatible transfusion
   (ii) Pregnancy
   (iii) Administration of horse serum or bacterial antitoxins
5. Immune anti-Rh antibodies result from:
   (i)   Previous incompatible transfusion
   (ii) Pregnancy (due to placental passage of fetal cells into maternal circulation)

Table 18.1   Blood products

Component	Description	Indications	ABO compatibility required	Cross-match required
Whole blood	450 ml Hct 0.35–0.45	Massive haemorrhage (>50% blood volume)	Yes	Yes
Plasma reduced blood with O A S e.g. SAG(M)	200 ml RBC with optimal additive solution (improving shelf life) Hct 0.5–0.7	Anaemia, bleeding Not recommended for neonates	Yes	Yes
Packed cells	200 ml RBC Hct 0.55–0.75	Anaemia, bleeding	Yes	Yes
Platelet concentrate	4 units pooled or single donor apheresis platelets (300 ml) Stored at 20°C 5-day shelf life	Bleeding due to thrombocytopenia or platelet dysfunction. Prophylaxis if platelets $< 20 \times 10^9/l$	Yes	No
Fresh frozen plasma (FFP)	50(paediatric) –250 ml packs	Deficiency of multiple coagulation factors	Yes	No
Cryoprecipitate	10–20 ml per unit Adult dose 6–20 u Rich in VIII and fibrinogen	Treatment of von Willebrand's disease and haemophilia A Bleeding due to low fibrinogen Treatment of DIC	Yes	No
Human albumin solution (HAS)				
4.5% purified protein fraction (PPF)	*100 ml* 4.5 g protein 16 mmol Na	Acute blood volume replacement Rx burns, acute pancreatitis, and as exchange fluid in plasmapheresis	No	No
20% salt-poor albumin	*100 ml* 15–25 g protein Up to 15 mmol Na Hyperosmotic, ∴ risk of pulmonary oedema	Short-term management of hypoproteinaemic patients with diuretic -resistant fluid overload, e.g. liver disease, nephrotic syndrome	No	No

Typing and crossmatching

1. Recipient serum must be screened for red cell antibodies prior to transfusion. If positive, full antibody identification should follow, with selection of blood lacking the appropriate antigen(s) for compatibility testing and transfusion
2. Whenever possible ABO and Rh(D) identical blood should be selected for recipients; if this is not available ABO Rh(D) compatible blood should be used.
   Note: Only 'lysin-free' (serum free of lytic anti-A or B) Group O donors can be considered as safe 'universal' donors

Administration

1. It is essential to check that crossmatched blood is for the recipient in question; failure to identify donor or recipient correctly is the main cause of transfusion-related morbidity/death
2. One unit of packed cells may be tranfused in about 90 minutes; slower transfusion with diuretic cover required in cases of previous/incipient heart failure
3. Careful regular observation of clinical condition of recipient, flow rate and i.v. site
4. One unit increases Hb level by approximately 1 g/dl

Indications/contraindications

1. Each patient's requirements must be considered in relation to age and mobility
2. Patients with *chronic* mild/moderate anaemia (Hb > 9 g/dl) usually compensate well and do not necessarily require blood
3. Patients with low-affinity haemoglobins, e.g. homozygous sickle cell anaemia, usually compensate well and may only require transfusion during crises
4. Unless very severe, readily corrected anaemias, such as PA/iron deficiency, are not indications for transfusion

Complications

Untoward reactions, usually minor, occur in about 5% of recipients:

1. Haemolytic—due to premature destruction of donor RBC by immune antibodies in recipient.
   Immediate:
   (i) Usually due to blood group incompatibility caused by clerical or administrative error. Preventable with fastidious adherence to standard procedures. Fatal in up to 10% cases
   (ii) Less frequently caused by immune RBC antibodies
   (iii) Early clinical features—apprehension, tachycardia, pyrexia, lumbar and chest pain, flushing, headache and nausea. Hypotension and shock may develop

   (iv) Sequelae:
      a. Intravascular haemolysis—haemoglobinaemia and haemoglobinuria
      b. Hyperbilirubinaemia and jaundice
      c. Oliguria and acute renal failure may supervene
      d. Haemorrhagic diathesis (reflecting DIC)—unusual
   (v) Treatment:
      a. Stop transfusion immediately
      b. Maintain blood volume, blood pressure and urinary output
      c. Send blood samples for DCT, repeat antibody screen and compatibility testing against transfused units. Pre-transfusion sample should be re-tested simultaneously
      d. Check FBC, platelet count, coagulation profile, renal function and tests for intravascular haemolysis

Delayed:
   (i) Unpredictable, and of variable severity
   (ii) Occurs in patients previously sensitised to RBC antigens by pregnancy or transfusion
   (iii) Pre-transfusion antibody screening negative
   (iv) Transfusion of blood carrying appropriate antigen stimulates a secondary anamnestic immune response within 7–10 days
   (v) Clinical features include fever, jaundice and anaemia with suboptimal increment in Hb for the quantity of blood transfused
   (vi) Underlines importance of repeating antibody screen if transfusion has been given > 48 hours previously and further blood is required
   (vii) Investigations—as for immediate haemolytic reactions
2. Non-haemolytic febrile transfusion reactions (NHFTR):
   (i) Due to leucocyte (HLA or neutrophil) or platelet antibodies stimulated by previous transfusion or pregnancy
   (ii) Fever usually occurs 30 min– 2 h after the start of transfusion
   (iii) Symptoms include feeling cold and shivery, rigors, apprehension, headache, flushing and nausea
   (iv) Temperature settles within a few hours
   (v) Treatment—slow or stop transfusion and treat symptomatically, e.g. with antipyretics, antihistamines ± steroids
   (vi) Check HLA (lymphocytotoxic) and neutrophil antibodies, and platelet-specific antibodies
   (vii) Recurrence is avoided by using leucocyte-depleted blood— by centrifugation and removal of buffy coat layer, filtration or using frozen-thawed washed RBC
3. Allergic:
   (i) Due to plasma protein antibodies, frequently anti-IgA in IgA deficient recipients

    (ii) Clinical features—usually urticaria with itching, pyrexia, headache and nausea. Rarely anaphylactic shock

    (iii) Treatment—stop or slow transfusion; antihistamines, occasionally steroids/adrenaline

    (iv) Prevention—prophylactic antihistamines pre-transfusion. Occasionally washed RBC required

4. Transmission of infection (largely preventable by careful donor screening):
    (i) Hepatitis B*
    (ii) Hepatitis C*
    (iii) Human immunodeficiency viruses—$HIV_1 \rightarrow$ AIDS*
                                      HIV_2
    (iv) Cytomegalovirus (fresh blood and granulocytes)
    (v) Syphilis*(spirochaetes can survive about 4 days in banked blood)
    (vi) Malaria (parasites viable for days/weeks)
    (vii) Brucellosis
    * Mandatory screening of donors in developed countries

5. Miscellaneous:
    (i) Post-transfusion purpura—related to development of PL^{A1} antibodies in previously sensitised PL^{A1}-negative recipients (see p.131)

    (ii) Infected blood:
        a. May give febrile reactions due to bacterial pyrogens (very rare), or septicaemia and collapse with high mortality due to Gram-negative organisms, e.g. coliforms, *Pseudomonas*. Symptoms and signs resemble those of ABO incompatibility. Requires i.v. broad-spectrum antibiotics
        b. Preventable by careful aseptic techniques in blood donation, storage in correct controlled conditions, use within 24 hours if open methods used in preparation

    (iii) Circulatory overload:
        a. Typically in elderly, chronically anaemic patients, but also in pregnant women and severely anaemic patients
        b. Clinical features—dyspnoea, cyanosis, pulmonary oedema
        c. Treatment—diuretics and slowing of transfusion rate. Emergency venesection is required exceptionally
        d. Prevention—use of packed cells, diuretic cover, and careful clinical monitoring

    (iv) Thrombophlebitis—in relation to drip site
    (v) Citrate toxicity—(with massive transfusions and impaired clearance)—causes hypocalcaemia
    (vi) Haemosiderosis—seen in patients who are chronically transfusion-dependent, e.g. in thalassaemia major. 'Symptomatic' after 100 units assuming no chelation (each

unit of blood contains 200 mg iron; maximum excretion rate is 1 mg/d)

PLATELETS

1. Typing
(i)   ABO and Rh (D) compatibility—ideal but not essential. Platelets of a different ABO group may cause a positive DCT (but rarely haemolysis) in recipient
(ii) HLA compatibility—ideal, usually impractical (1 in 4 chance of HLA identity among a patient's siblings). May be necessary for patients with refractory thrombocytopenia and lymphocytotoxic antibodies

2. Preparation
(i)   From fresh whole blood donations stored at room temperature, with separation by centrifugation as soon as possible after donation
(ii) Single donor apheresis unit (equivalent to 4–6 units prepared as in (i)). For patients requiring 'special' platelets—e.g. HLA-matched, CMV-negative
(iii) Frozen in dimethylsulfoxide or glycerol—normal post-transfusion survival
(iv) Storage—at room temperature on a rotator. Storage life now 5–7 days using 'extended storage' polyolefin packs which allow efficient gaseous exchange.
(v)   Administration—as single donor apheresis pack, or as pooled platelet concentrates from 4–6 donors

3. Indications
(i)   Prophylaxis in the presence of very low platelet counts ($< 20 \times 10^9$/l) if likely to be transient, e.g. following chemotherapy
(ii) Symptomatic thrombocytopenia, i.e. bleeding:
   a. In haematological malignancies—especially in chemotherapy-induced marrow suppression
   b. In severe aplastic anaemia—see p.52
   c. In disorders of platelet function
   d. In life-threatening haemorrhage associated with ITP (platelet survival is often reduced and the therapeutic gain transient)

4. Complications
(i)   Development of alloantibodies—may cause adverse reactions in recipient and platelet refractoriness
(ii) Infective risk—hepatitis B and C

GRANULOCYTES

1. Typing
(i)   ABO and Rh compatability—a minimum requirement
(ii) HLA compatability—desirable. Donors are often close relatives of the recipient

2. Preparation
(i)   Continuous flow centrifugal (CFC) systems—white cells are separated by differential density centrifugation
(ii) Yields may be improved by prior administration of corticosteroids to the donor and addition of hydroxyethyl starch or gelatin (sedimenting agents) to the blood

3. Administration
(i)   The minimum number of cells necessary for clinical effectiveness is not certain—probably at least 4×10^{10} granulocytes daily for 3–4 days
(iii) Cells should be given as soon as possible (function deteriorates on storage)

4. Indications
In life threatening localised infections in neutropenic patients not responding to antibiotics.
Note: The criteria for transfusions require better definition (empiric or prophylactic use is still controversial).

5. Complications (in recipients)
Most serious is ARDS due to aggregates in lungs. Development of leucocyte antibodies, reactions and CMV transmission (unless CMV negative donors used).

AUTOLOGOUS TRANSFUSION

Three main types:
1. Predeposit—blood taken from recipient in advance of planned transfusion (usually for surgical procedure) and stored until needed. It is possible to collect up to 5 units on a weekly basis with storage life of 35 days at 4°C
2. Isovolaemic haemodilution—blood taken immediately prior to surgery (with volume replacement by colloid or crystalloid) to be reinfused at end of operation
3. Perioperative salvage—lost blood is collected, washed and reinfused using a mechanical 'cell-saver' during perioperative bleeding. Contraindicated in bowel and pancreatic surgery and surgery for malignancy

Advantages
1. Abolishes transfusion-related risks of infection and allo-immunisation
2. Provides useful source of blood (frozen) for patients with rare groups or with antibodies against high frequency RBC antigens, for whom it is impossible to obtain compatible blood at short notice
3. Isovolaemic haemodilution improves rheological properties of blood by reducing viscosity
4. Conserves supplies of standard donor blood

Disadvantages
1. Relatively expensive and time consuming; requires careful organisation
2. Requires advance planning with cooperation of surgeons to confirm definite dates at least one month in advance of surgery
3. Applicable to a limited population
4. Appropriate for relatively few surgical procedures
5. Those patients most likely to benefit, e.g. multitransfused, are those least likely to be suitable donors for autologous transfusion

TRANSFUSION FOR MASSIVE BLOOD LOSS

Massive blood loss may be defined as blood loss requiring transfusion equivalent to total blood volume in less than 24 hours.
1. Treat hypotension promptly, maintaining a urine output of ≥ 30 ml/h by infusing:
    (i) crystalloids (saline, Ringer's lactate) or
    (ii) colloids (hydroxyethyl starch or gelatin) up to 40% blood volume (2–3 litres), after which 4.5% human albumin solution should be used to maintain colloid osmotic pressure
    Note: Blood samples for crossmatching should be taken before infusing colloids
2. ABO Rh(D) specific blood should be used, unless in extreme emergencies when Group O blood can be used initially, followed by ABO specific blood. Grouping and crossmatching should be completed within 15 minutes in emergencies
3. Platelets (one unit per 10 kg body weight) should be infused if the platelet count is $< 50 \times 10^9/l$ or falling (between 50 and $100 \times 10^9/l$). Platelet function may be impaired in massively transfused or traumatised patients
4. Fresh frozen plasma should be given if PT or APTT/KCCT is prolonged ($> 1.5 \times$ normal), though there is generally a poor correlation between in vitro abnormality and clinical bleeding diathesis. Cryoprecipitate is a rich source of fibrinogen, VIII and vWF

5. Packed cells and cells in optimal additive solutions are satisfactory for initial resuscitation, but if massive transfusion is required, the use of whole blood, preferably less than 7 days old (less deterioration in terms of reduced O_2 affinity, increased plasma potassium and microaggregate formation) is more satisfactory and economical
6. For massive, uncontrolled haemorrhage requiring surgical treatment, whole blood, packed cells, colloids and crystalloids should be used to maintain blood volume, reserving plasma and platelets until haemorrhage is controlled
7. Component therapy with plasma and platelets is indicated when bleeding is presumed due to deficient haemostasis rather than from major blood vessels

FURTHER ADVANCED READING

Contreras M, Hewitt P 1989 Clinical blood transfusion. In: Hoffbrand A V, Lewis S M (eds) Postgraduate haematology. Heinemann, London, pp 269–293

Mollison P L, Engelfriet C P, Contreras M 1987 Blood transfusion in clinical medicine, 8th edn. Blackwell, Oxford

United Kingdom Health Departments 1989 Handbook of transfusion medicine. HMSO, London

19. Haematopoiesis, normal and abnormal

Stem cell concepts
1. Pluripotent stem cells (0.01–0.05 per cent of total marrow cell population):
   (i)   Produce more stem cells (self-renewal)
   (ii) Produce:
         a. Lymphoid stem cells
         b. Multipotent colony-forming cells/units (CFC/CFU) of mixed potential capable of differentiating into mature cells of the myeloid series
         c. More developmentally-restricted cells including a range of unipotent CFC/CFU
   (iii) Ultimately differentiate to produce mature cell types—erythrocytes, neutrophils, eosinophils, basophils, monocytes, macrophages, osteoclasts, T and B lymphocytes and platelets
2. Following depletion of marrow cells, secondary to chemotherapy/radiation, regeneration of haematopoiesis depends on proliferation and differentiation of cells from:
   a. Lineage-restricted progenitor cells—short-term renewal
   b. Pluripotent stem cells—longer-term renewal
3. Fundamental defects will affect the range of cell lines, resulting in multi-lineage lympho-myelodysplasia

Haemopoietic growth factors
Glycoproteins with polypeptide chains of similar length and high biological activity; produced by more than one cell type:
1. As a result of in vitro cell culture studies, an increasing number of factors which can initiate and promote the development of colony forming cells/units (CFC/CFU) have been identified
2. Recombinant DNA technology has resulted in the isolation of genes coding for these colony-stimulating factors (CSFs) and the ability to produce large quantities (using bacterial, yeast or mammalian cell systems)
3. CSFs have distinct structures at the molecular level and there are specific receptors on the surface of the 'target cells'

4. Erythropoietin (Epo)—a hormone, production of which by the juxtatubular cells of the kidney is regulated by tissue oxygen tension; principal stimulus for terminal maturation of erythroid precursors
5. Some interleukins (IL) which modulate proliferation and differentiation of lymphoid cells also have important effects on myeloid cell precursors
6. Two or more growth factors are usually required for optimal regulation of precursor differentiation, e.g. erythropoietin and GM-CSF/IL-3 for erythroid differentiation. The interactions of growth factors are very complex; there are many examples of synergy and inhibitory effects also occur
7. The microenvironment of the bone marrow—stem cells, the various precursors, stromal cells, fibroblasts and endothelial cells in close relationship provide the milieu in which cell-factor–cell interactions take place
8. The cellular origin and sites of action of the various growth factors, largely deduced from in vitro studies, are shown in Figure 19.1

Clinical use of haemopoietic growth factors
1. Experience is accumulating on the in vivo effects of the various colony stimulating factors, principally GM-CSF and G-CSF:
   (i)   To reduce the morbidity of chemotherapy—duration of neutropenia can be considerably reduced and thereby the risk of infection
   (ii) To allow intensification of chemotherapy—dose escalation and/or reduction in intervals between treatment
   (iii) To stimulate marrow function following bone marrow transplantation
   (iv) To stimulate marrow function in bone marrow/peripheral blood haemopoietic cell donors (pre-transplant)
   (v)   In treatment of cyclical neutropenia
   (vi) In recruiting quiescent leukaemic cells into cell cycle enhancing sensitivity to cytotoxic drugs
   (vii) In treatment of myelodysplastic syndromes (leukaemic transformation is a risk)
2. Recombinant erythropoietin (Epo) is being used increasingly in patients with severe anaemia due to end-stage renal disease
3. The synthesis of the various interleukins is being followed by formulation for clinical use and exploration of their therapeutic rôles
4. The scope for future advances in 'biological therapy' with the range of growth factors (and also growth inhibitory molecules) is very considerable

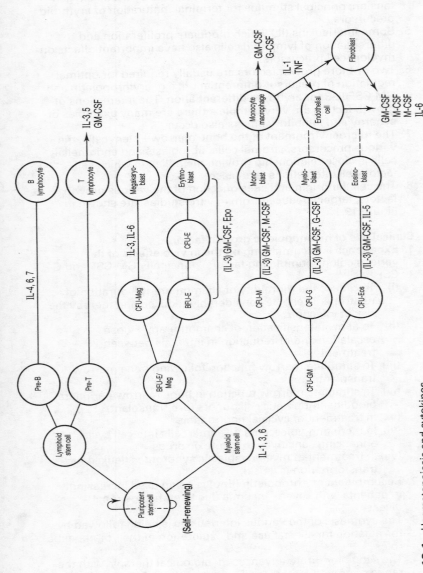

Fig. 19.1 Haematopoiesis and cytokines

Erythropoiesis

1. Basic changes in normoblastic erythropoiesis
(i)   Reduction in cell size and nuclear-cytoplasmic ratio
(ii) Nuclear maturation—nucleoli are lost, chromatin clumps and the small pyknotic nucleus is eventually extruded

2. Nomenclature
— Erythroblast
— Pronormoblast
— Polychromatic normoblast
— Orthochromic normoblast
— Reticulocyte
— Mature red cell (Erythrocyte)

3. Modulating factors
(i)   Erythropoietin
(ii) Other hormones:
     a. Stimulatory—androgens, thyroxine, growth hormone
     b. Inhibitory—oestrogens, progesterone
(iii) CSFs
(iv) Haematinics:
     a. availability of iron has an important influence on the number of cell divisions
     b. B_{12} and folate status

4. Haemoglobin synthesis
(i)   Globin chains:
     a. Synthesised by polysomes in the erythroblast cytoplasm
     b. Amino-acid sequence is determined by DNA-coded genetic information
     c. Two pairs of polypeptide chains are formed normally:
(ii) Haem—see Fig. 19.2

		% in normal adult
Hb. GOWER	$\alpha_2\epsilon_2$ (embryonic)	0
Hb-F	$\alpha_2\delta_2$ (fetal)	<2
Hb-A	$\alpha_2\beta_2$ (adult)	96+
Hb-A2	$\alpha_2\delta_2$ (adult)	1–3
Hb-GOWER exists in 2 forms (I & II):		
Hb-GOWER I	ϵ_4	
Hb-GOWER II	$\alpha_2\epsilon_2$	

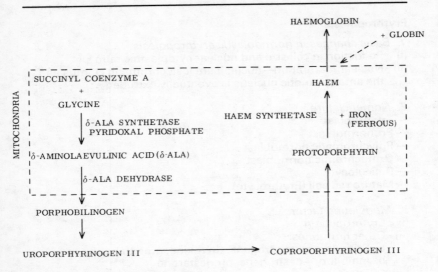

Fig. 19.2   Haem synthetic pathway

(iii) Haemoglobin molecules—normal production depends on the
normal synthesis of haem and globin chains which are inter-
related

Abnormal erythropoiesis
1. *Quantitative*—from aplasia to hyperplasia
2. *Qualitative* (with or without quantitative changes):
   (i) Ineffective, due to increased intramedullary haemolysis—the
   production of reticulocytes and mature red cells is
   inappropriate for the erythroid cell mass, e.g.
   thalassaemia
   (ii) Megaloblastic (also ineffective)—impaired DNA synthesis
   with delayed maturation of nucleus (see p.10)
   (iii) Sideroblastic change—the diagnostic feature is the
   disposition of iron (siderotic granules) in a ring around the
   nucleus of the red cell precursor. *Not* to be confused with the
   increase in siderotic granules *randomly* distributed in
   cytoplasm and commonly seen in many dyshaemopoietic
   states
   (iv) Vacuolation of erythroblasts:
       a. Irregular non-haemoglobinised areas in late precursors
       indicating defective haemoglobinisation, as in iron
       deficiency or impaired iron utilisation
       b. Clearly demarcated vacuoles at any stage of
       erythropoiesis, e.g. the alcohol effect
   (v) 'Dyserythropoiesis'—often applied to a variety of

abnormalities but should be reserved for erythropoiesis which shows:
  a. Atypical nuclei—multiple, multilobulated or fragmented
  b. Asynchronous nuclear/cytoplasmic maturation
Usually seen in the context of myelodysplastic syndromes (MDS)

Granulopoiesis
1. Basic changes in normal granulopoiesis:
   (i) Reduction in nuclear–cytoplasmic ratio
   (ii) Loss of nucleoli and clumping of nuclear chromatin
   (iii) The cytoplasm becomes less basophilic and granules appear (firstly 'primary' in the promyelocyte, then 'specific', determining the cell type—neutrophil, eosinophil or basophil)
   (iv) Indentation of nucleus and ultimately hypersegmentation
   (v) Development of motility and ability to phagocytose
2. Cell nomenclature:
   — Myeloblast
   — Promyeloblast
   — Myelocyte
   — Metamyelocyte
   — 'Stab'/'band' form
   — Segmented neutrophil
   (Eosinophils and basophils develop through equivalent steps with specific granules appearing at the myelocyte stage)
3. Modulating factors—cytokines

Abnormal granulopoiesis
1. *Quantitative*—from aplasia to hyperplasia
2. *Qualitative*:
   (i) Ineffective myelopoiesis or maturation arrest
   (ii) Megaloblastic (also ineffective) – the giant metamyelocyte and the hypersegmented polymorph are of diagnostic importance
   (iii) Dysplastic as in MDS
   (iv) Malignant, as in the myeloid leukaemias

Thrombopoiesis
1. Basic changes in normal thrombopoiesis:
   (i) Nuclear division without cell division
   (ii) Daughter nuclei form a large lobulated nuclear mass
   (iii) The cytoplasm increases
   (iv) Cytoplasmic azurophilic granules appear
2. Cell nomenclature:
   — Megakaryoblast
   — Promegakaryocyte
   — Megakaryocyte

3. Platelet production—platelets are formed as sub-units of the megakaryocyte cytoplasm and subsequently released
4. Modulating factors—cytokines

Abnormal thrombopoiesis

1. *Quantitative* —from absence of megakaryocytes to excess
2. *Qualitative*:
    (i)   Ineffective
    (ii) Megaloblastic (also ineffective)—abnormal megakaryocytes with hypersegmented nuclei
    (iii) Dysplastic as in MDS
    (iv) Malignant

20. Bone marrow examination

Examination of bone marrow is frequently carried out as part of a haematological investigation, though this should not be done before assessment of the peripheral blood indices and film or without clear indication.

Aspirate
1. Using wide-bore needle with adjustable guard (e.g. Salah, Klima) under local anaesthesia
2. Sternal or iliac crest specimens are usually obtained
3. Films are routinely assessed for:
   (i)   Cellularity
   (ii) Erythropoiesis
   (iii) Granulopoiesis
   (iv) Thrombopoiesis
   (v)   Presence of excess plasma/blast cells
   (vi) Presence of atypical cells, malignant cells
   (vii) Sideroblast population (normal/abnormal) and iron stores (ferrocyanide stain)
4. In some cases, e.g. leukaemia, additional preparations for cytochemistry, immunological marker studies and cytogenetics are required
5. 'Dry' or 'blood' tap — failure to obtain marrow tissue may be due to:
   (i)   Fibrosis, e.g. myelofibrosis
   (ii) Dense infiltration with malignant cells (haematological, as in leukaemias, or non-haematological, as in carcinomatosis)
   (iii) Faulty technique
   'Touch preparations' obtained at trephine biopsy may be helpful in such cases

Trephine biopsy
1. A variety of instruments have been used but the Islam or Jamshidi needles have the merit of being:
   (i)   Easy to use with minimal trauma and under local anaesthesia without special facilities

    (ii) Capable of providing adequate material for
          histopathological assessment
2. Histopathological assessment:
    (i) *Quantitative*—haemopoietic tissue in relation to bone, fat,
        reticulin; relative proportions of cell types
    (ii) *Qualitative/quantitative*—diagnosis and classification, e.g.
        of haematological and non-haematological malignancies,
        confirmation of myeloproliferative disease

21. Red cell function— oxygen transport

Basic concepts

1. The principal function of haemoglobin is to carry oxygen to the tissues
2. The oxygen affinity of haemoglobin is influenced by various factors:
   - (i) pH and CO_2 — acidosis decreases O_2 affinity (Bohr effect)
   - (ii) Temperature — increase results in decreased O_2 affinity
   - (iii) Levels of the glycolytic intermediate 2, 3-diphosphoglycerate (2, 3-DPG) in red cells — increase produces decrease in O_2 affinity
   - (iv) Oxyhaemoglobin has a high affinity, deoxyhaemoglobin a low affinity for oxygen
   - (v) 2, 3-DPG binds to the deoxy form, between the β chains, tending to maintain haemoglobin in a low affinity state
3. The oxygen affinity is of critical importance in the uptake of oxygen in the lungs and the release of oxygen in the tissues

Clinical significance

1. Anaemia:
   - (i) Reduced oxygen affinity of haemoglobin reflects increase in red cell 2, 3-DPG due to hypoxia
   - (ii) Enhanced release of oxygen to the tissues tends to compensate for anaemia (explains the lack of symptoms in many chronic anaemias)
2. Hypoxia in heart disease, thyrotoxicosis and at high altitudes — increases in 2, 3-DPG tend to compensate, reducing the requirement for increased cardiac output
3. Acid-base disturbance, e.g. in diabetic acidosis:
   - (i) 2, 3-DPG is reduced but any tendency to increase in oxygen affinity is offset by the Bohr effect
   - (ii) The Bohr effect is immediate; 2, 3-DPG adjustment slower (over several hours)
   - (iii) Rapid correction of acidosis is therefore undesirable (sudden increases in oxygen affinity may impair tissue oxygenation)
4. Hypoxia with acid-base change — Factors affecting affinity may

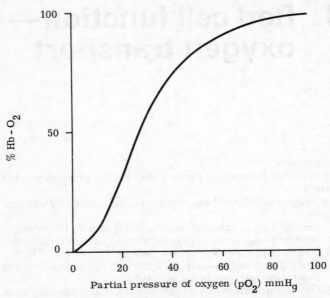

Fig. 21.1 Oxygen dissociation curve of adult whole blood (pH 7.4)

have an additive effect or tend to diminish the shifts in the oxygen dissociation curve

5. Red cell enzyme defects — Changes in 2, 3-DPG depend on the enzyme deficiency; e.g. in pyruvate kinase deficiency there is a build-up of preceding intermediates with increased 2, 3-DPG levels (patients tend to compensate well for anaemia)
6. Blood transfusion:
    (i)   2, 3-DPG levels fall in stored blood (especially in acid citrate dextrose, ACD)
    (ii) Correction takes many hours following transfusion into a recipient
    (iii) Of importance only when rapid, massive blood replacement is necessary.
    (iv) 2, 3-DPG levels can be maintained by optimal additive solutions, e.g. saline adenine glucose mannitol (SAGM), increasing the storage life of blood from 21 to 35 days

22. Neutrophil function —microbicidal activity

One of the important defences of the body against infection is the phagocytosis and killing of microorganisms by neutrophil polymorphs. The following are the principal aspects of the mechanism:

1. Stimulation of granulopoiesis — by colony stimulating factors, e.g. GM-CSF, G-CSF, M-CSF (see p.162)
2. Inflammation — neutrophils adhere to the endothelium of dilated capillaries
3. Migration and chemotaxis — neutrophils are attracted by:
   (i)   Substances released by phagocytosing cells and traumatised tissue
   (ii) Activated complement components
   (iii) Bacterial proteins
4. Phagocytosis:
   (i) Antibodies and antibody-activated complement components coat microorganisms and act as opsonins, facilitating phagocytosis
   (ii) The microorganisms are encircled by pseudopodia and become internalised in the phagocytic vacuole
5. Intracellular killing of microorganisms:
   (i)   Metabolic burst of oxidative metabolism leads to production of H_2O_2
   (ii) Granules from cytoplasmic lysosomes are discharged into the phagocytic vacuole
   (iii) A number of microbicidal systems are activated:
      a. Oxygen dependent — H_2O_2 + halide (e.g. iodine) ± myeloperoxidase; superoxide
      b. Oxygen independent — pH (acidic), lysozyme, lactoferrin and cationic proteins

Minor defects of these mechanisms are probably common in many disease states but their clinical relevance is often obscure (see p.101)

23. The haematological indices

RED CELL INDICES

Basic concepts

1. The normal ranges are usually derived from Gaussian distribution curves
2. Methodology influences the normal values:
   - (i) Most laboratories use electronic counters in which packed cell volume (PCV) is derived from red cell count (RBC) and mean cell volume (MCV) (1.5–3% *lower* than values obtained by centrifugal microhaematocrit methods)
3. The following may be determined by calculation using measurements made by electronic counters:
   - (i) Packed cell volume (PCV or haematocrit)

$$\frac{RBC \times MCV}{1000} \qquad (RBC, \times 10^{12}/l; \; MCV, \; fl)$$

   - (ii) Mean corpuscular haemoglobin (MCH), i.e. mean *weight* of haemoglobin in cell

$$\frac{Haemoglobin \; level \; (Hb) \times 10}{RBC} \qquad pg \; (Hb, \; g/dl)$$

   - (iii) Mean corpuscular haemoglobin concentration (MCHC), i.e. mean *concentration* of haemoglobin in the red cells

$$\frac{Hb}{PCV} \qquad g/dl$$

      Note: Reduction in MCHC (e.g. in iron deficiency anaemia) is less marked when calculated from electronic counts than when derived from Hb and micro-haematocrit, where trapped plasma causes an appreciable error

4. The clinician is usually presented with a full range of electronically determined indices which are generally very reliable and for which there are standard quality controls

Normal red cell indices

Haemoglobin level (Hb)	men	13.0–18.0 g/dl
	women	11.5–16.5 g/dl
Packed cell volume (PCV)	men	0.40–0.54
	women	0.37–0.47
Red cell count (RBC)	men	$4.5–6.5 \times 10^{12}$/l
	women	$3.8–5.8 \times 10^{12}$/l
Mean corpuscular volume (MCV)		78–96 fl
Mean corpuscular haemoglobin (MCH)		27–32 pg
Mean corpuscular haemoglobin concentration (MCHC)		31–35 g/dl

These values correspond to values quoted in standard reference works. They are intended as a practical guide but account must be taken of methodology in the close interpretation of minor changes. Indices for adults are given; values for infants and children may be obtained from the standard reference works

Additional normal values
Reticulocytes (visual counts of supravitally stained blood film) 0.2–2.0%

Red cell volume (or mass)	(isotopic determinations)	men	25–35 ml/kg
		women	20–30 ml/kg
Plasma volume			40–50 ml/kg
Total blood volume			60–80 ml/kg

Clinical aspects
1. Hb, PCV and, to a lesser extent, RBC are used in assessing degrees of anaemia or polycythaemia but may mislead due to increase or decrease in plasma volume, overhydration/dehydration (the red cell volume/mass is required to confirm true polycythaemia)
2. Although the assessment 'microcytic', 'normocytic' or 'macrocytic' is often based on the MCV, there may be considerable variation from the mean, which can be seen in the blood film
3. The fact that indices are readily available has resulted in the early diagnosis of subtle haematological abnormalities
   Examples:
   (i) The low MCV with little or no reduction in Hb in thalassaemia trait
   (ii) The raised MCV with normal Hb in some patients with B_{12}/folate deficiency
   (iii) The slightly increased MCV in alcoholism and MDS

4. An important source of 'error' may result from agglutination of red cells, e.g. in cold agglutinin-associated conditions, RBC is falsely low and MCV falsely high

WHITE CELL INDICES

Total leucocyte count (WBC)
Now routinely obtained using electronic counters.

Differential leucocyte count
1. Electronically determined by 'gating' (Coulter) or by optical flow cytometry (Technicon). Manual differentials are obtained by counting at least 100 cells visually in a blood film
2. Percentages of various types of white cells are often quoted but in defining abnormalities clearly, *absolute* numbers should be calculated

Normal values

Total	leucocyte count (WBC)	$4.0-11.0 \times 10^9/l$
	neutrophils	$2.0-7.5 \times 10^9/l$ (40–50%)
	lymphocytes	$1.5-4.0 \times 10^9/l$ (20–45%)
	monocytes	$0.2-0.8 \times 10^9/l$ (2–10%)
	eosinophils	$0.04-0.4 \times 10^9/l$ (1–6%)
	basophils	$0.01-0.1 \times 10^9/l$ (< 1%)

PLATELET COUNTS

Now routinely by electronic counters. One source of inaccuracy results from the reduction of platelets in the blood sample because of inadequate anticoagulation with clot formation, e.g. due to overfilled sample bottles. Platelet clumping is another possible cause of error.

Normal values: $150-400 \times 10^9/l$

COAGULATION TESTS

Bleeding time (BT)— duration of bleeding following standard punctures of the skin, e.g. by template method.

Normal range: 2.5–9.5 min for Simplate II template

Hess test or capillary resistance test (CRT)— number of petechiae within a 3 cm diameter area below the cubital fossa after 5-min inflation of a sphygmomanometer cuff (at between systolic and diastolic pressure). A relatively crude test.

Normal: <5

One-stage prothrombin time (PT)—clotting time of citrated plasma to which thromboplastin and calcium have been added. Abnormal in Factor V, VII, X, prothrombin and fibrinogen deficiencies (and in patients on oral anticoagulants where it is used in monitoring dosage).

Normal range: 12–15 s (*but* a normal control must be tested concurrently because of variability). Standardisation by use of INR (see p.147)

Activated partial thromboplastin time, (APTT) or kaolin-cephalin clotting time (KCT)—clotting time of citrated plasma accelerated by addition of a clotting factor activator (kaolin), phospholipid and calcium. Sensitive test of factors V, VIII, IX, X, XI, XII, prothrombin and fibrinogen deficiencies. Used to monitor heparin therapy.

Normal values: e.g. 30–45 s (again, comparison with normal control is essential)

Thrombin time—clotting time of plasma to which thrombin has been added (thereby converting fibrinogen to fibrin). Abnormal in presence of heparin and fibrin/fibrinogen degradation products and in dysfibrinogenaemia or fibrinogen depletion.

Other tests—include assays of coagulation factors, fibrinogen and fibrin degradation products (FDP) and the tests of platelet function. Further description of coagulation tests, their application and normal values may be obtained from the standard reference works.

24. Blood film abnormalities

RED CELL ABNORMALITIES

1. Size
(i) Microcytosis—e.g. in iron deficiency anaemia, thalassaemia
(ii) Macrocytosis—e.g. in megaloblastic anaemia, liver disease
(iii) Anisocytosis—exaggerated variation in size, e.g. in iron deficiency anaemia responding to treatment

2. Shape
(i) Poikilocytosis—deviation from normal shape, e.g. elongated pencil-like forms in iron deficiency anaemia, tear-shaped forms in myelofibrosis
(ii) Specific 'diagnostic' forms:
    a. Spherocyte—e.g. in hereditary spherocytosis
    b. Elliptocyte—e.g. in hereditary elliptocytosis
    c. Sickle cell—e.g. in sickle cell anaemia (HbSS)
    d. Acanthocyte—irregularly spiny/spiculated cells, e.g. in abetalipoproteinaemia
    e. Burr/spur cell/schistocyte—the result of cell fragmentation, e.g. in DIC, uraemia
    f. Stomatocyte—invaginated cell (cup-shaped in wet preparations), e.g. in hereditary stomatocytosis, liver disease

3. Haemoglobinisation/staining
(i) Anisochromia—exaggerated variation in colour—(i.e. in pinkness with Romanowsky stains), e.g. in iron deficiency anaemia responding to treatment
(ii) Hypochromia—pallor, typically centrally, e.g. in iron deficiency anaemia
(iii) Polychromasia—diffuse bluish cytoplasmic tint, due to RNA, denoting prematurity (may be seen as reticulocytes with appropriate stain), increased with increased erythropoiesis, e.g. in haemolytic states
(iv) Specific 'diagnostic' forms:
    a. 'Target-cell' ('Mexican hat' or leptocyte)—hypochromic cell

with central 'blob' and peripheral ring of haemoglobinisation, due to decreased cell thickness (e.g. in iron deficiency and thalassaemia) and/or increased cell surface area (e.g. in obstructive jaundice)
b. Stomatocyte—mouth-like unstained area (corresponding to the invagination)

4. Inclusions

(i)   Punctate basophilia (basophilic stippling) — fine dark blue granules; due to RNA (reticulocytes) iron (siderocytes) *or* globin chains as in thalassaemia
(ii) Howell–Jolly bodies—round densely staining particles representing nuclear remnants containing DNA, e.g. post-splenectomy, megaloblastic anaemia
(iii) Siderotic granules (in siderocytes)—ferric iron not utilised in haem synthesis, showing positive Prussian blue reaction (with ferrocyanide) e.g. post-splenectomy, lead poisoning
(iv) Reticulum/fine granules (in reticulocytes)—RNA in immature cells precipitated by supra-vital dyes
(v)   H bodies—numerous blue granules (supra-vital stain) due to precipitated haemoglobin as in HbH disease (α thalassaemia)
(vi) Heinz bodies—rounded/irregular large granules (supra-vital stain) usually solitary, due to precipitated globin–glutathione complexes as in unstable haemoglobinopathies (e.g. Hb Zurich) and as an oxidant drug effect

GRANULOCYTE (POLYMORPHONUCLEAR) ABNORMALITIES

1. Nuclear

(i)   Macropolycyte—large hypersegmented neutrophil, the nucleus with 6+ lobes, due to abnormal granulopoiesis as in megaloblastic anaemia
(ii) Pelger–Hüet anomaly—bilobed 'dumb-bell' nucleus due to defective segmentation, hereditary (autosomal dominant) or acquired, e.g. in acute myeloblastic leukaemias, myelodysplasia

2. Cytoplasmic

(i)   Hypogranularity/agranularity—due to reduction in specific granules/absence of all granules (and therefore enzymes), e.g. in acute myeloblastic leukaemias, myelodysplasia
(ii) 'Toxic' granulation—coarse granulation, e.g. in infection
(iii) Specific 'diagnostic' types—e.g. giant granules in the hereditary Chediak–Higashi syndrome

LYMPHOCYTE/MONONUCLEAR CELL ABNORMALITIES

1. 'Atypical lymphocytes'—covers a variety of forms, larger than normal, often with abundant pale vacuolated cytoplasm and irregular outline, e.g. in infectious mononucleosis, a variety of viral infections, some malignant haematological diseases
2. Large granular lymphocytes (LGLs)—T suppressor cells with natural killer activity. Found as benign association with rheumatoid arthritis and Felty's syndrome, but may herald a malignant lymphoproliferative disorder
3. 'Smear' or 'basket' cells—naked lymphocytic nuclei divested of cytoplasm, typically in CLL
4. Hairy-cell—larger than normal lymphocyte with irregular cytoplasmic projections, pathognomonic of hairy-cell leukaemia
5. Sézary cell—large lymphoid 'T' cell with abundant pale blue cytoplasm and cerebriform nucleus as in Sézary syndrome, mycosis fungoides
6. Malignant lymphoid cells—variably atypical cells, some with nuclear clefting or nucleoli, may be seen in malignant lymphomas
7. Prolymphocyte of prolymphocytic leukaemia—large lymphoid cell with large vesicular nucleolus but relatively well condensed nuclear chromatin
8. Türk cell—similar to a plasma cell, round/oval, usually with an eccentric nucleus and deeply basophilic cytoplasm, e.g. in viral infections such as rubella

PLATELET ABNORMALITIES

Macrothrombocytes—larger than normal; increased numbers may reflect:
1. Increased thrombopoiesis, e.g. in blood loss, inflammatory states
2. Disordered thrombopoiesis, e.g. myeloproliferative diseases, when giant/bizarre forms may be seen
3. Post-splenectomy state

Appendix

CLASSIFICATION OF NON-HODGKIN'S LYMPHOMAS

Working formulation	Kiel equivalent or related terms

Low-grade

A. Malignant Lymphoma
   Small lymphocytic
      consistent with CLL   ML lymphocytic, CLL
      plasmacytoid   ML lymphoplasmacytic/
                                   lymphoplasmacytoid

B. Malignant Lymphoma, follicular
   Predominantly small cleaved cell
      diffuse areas,
      sclerosis

                              ML centroblastic-
                              centrocytic (small),
                              follicular ± diffuse

C. Malignant Lymphoma, follicular
   Mixed, small cleaved and
   large cell
      diffuse areas,
      sclerosis

Intermediate-grade

D. Malignant Lymphoma, follicular
   Predominantly large cell   ML centroblastic-centrocytic
      diffuse areas,   (large), follicular ± diffuse
      sclerosis

E. Malignant Lymphoma, diffuse
   Small cleaved cell,   ML centrocytic (small)
      sclerosis

F. Malignant Lymphoma, diffuse   ML centroblastic-centrocytic
   Mixed, small and large cell,   (small), diffuse
      sclerosis;   ML lymphoplasmacytic/
      epithelioid cell component   -cytoid, polymorphic

G. Malignant Lymphoma, diffuse   ML centroblastic-centrocytic
   Large cell   (large), diffuse
      cleaved cell   ML centrocytic (large)
      non-cleaved cell   ML centroblastic
      sclerosis

Working formulation	Kiel equivalent or related terms
High-grade	
H. Malignant Lymphoma	
Large cell, immunoblastic	ML immunoblastic
plasmacytoid	
clear cell	
polymorphous	T-zone lymphoma
epithelioid cell component	Lymphoepithelioid cell lymphoma
I. Malignant lymphoma	
Lymphoblastic	
convoluted cell	ML lymphoblastic, convoluted cell type
non-convoluted cell	ML lymphoblastic, unclassified
J. Malignant Lymphoma	
Small non-cleaved cell	
Burkitt's	
follicular areas	ML lymphoblastic, Burkitt type and other B-lymphoblastic
Miscellaneous	
Composite	—
Mycosis fungoides	Mycosis fungoides
Histiocytic	—
Extramedullary plasmacytoma	ML plasmacytic
Unclassifiable	—
Other	—

Recommended text books and reference works

General references

Firkin F, Chestermann C, Pennington D, Rush B 1989 De Gruchy's clinical haematology in medical practice. 5th edn, Blackwell, Oxford

Hann I, Gibson J, Letsky E A 1991 Fetal and neonatal haematology. Baillière Tindall, London

Hoffbrand A V (ed) 1988 Recent advances in haematology 5. Churchill Livingstone, Edinburgh

Hoffbrand A V, Lewis S M (eds) 1989 Postgraduate haematology, 3rd edn. Heinemann, Oxford

Nathan D G, Oski F A 1991 Hematology of childhood and infancy, 4th edn. W B Saunders, Philadelphia

Roberts B E (ed) 1991 Standard haematology practice. Blackwell, Oxford

Wiernik P H, Canellos G P, Kyle R A, Schiffer C A 1991 Neoplastic diseases of the blood. Churchill Livingstone, Edinburgh

Practical reference works

Chanarin I (ed) 1989 Laboratory haematology. An account of laboratory techniques. Churchill Livingstone, Edinburgh

Dacie J V, Lewis S M 1991 Practical haematology, 7th edn. Churchill Livingstone, Edinburgh

Atlases

Hoffbrand A V, Pettit J E 1987 Clinical haematology illustrated. An integrated text and colour atlas. Churchill Livingstone, Edinburgh

McDonald G, Paul J, Cruickshank B 1989 Atlas of haematology, 5th edn. Churchill Livingstone, Edinburgh

Recommended specialist journals

British Journal of Haematology
Blood
Blood Reviews
Clinics in Haematology
Clinical Haematology
Seminars in Haematology

Index